Reducing the Stigma of Mental Illness

The stigma attached to mental illness is the main obstacle to better mental health care and better quality of life for people who have the illness, for their families, for their communities and for health service staff who deal with psychiatric disorders. Stigma is pernicious and there are indications that, despite advances of psychiatry and medicine, it continues to grow and have more and often terrible consequences for patients and families.

In 1996, the WPA began an international programme to fight the stigma and discrimination associated with schizophrenia. The 'Open the Doors' programme has been implemented since then in more than 20 countries and has involved about 200 different anti-stigma interventions.

This book details the results of these international efforts and provides recommendations and guidance for those seeking to join this initiative or to start similar efforts for dispelling stigma and discrimination.

Norman Sartorius is one of the most prominent and influential psychiatrists of his generation. He has served as Director of the Division of Mental Health at the World Health Organization, and subsequently as President of the World Psychiatric Association. He is a member of the Council of the World Psychiatric Association and of the Expert Advisory Panel of the World Health Organization. He is an honorary professor of the University of London, a professor at the Universities of Zagreb and Prague and has held or holds professorial appointments at the Department of Psychiatry of the University of Geneva and at several other universities in Europe, the USA and China; he is a senior associate of the Faculty of the Johns Hopkins School of Public Health in Baltimore. He has written over 300 scientific papers and has authored, co-authored or edited more than 40 books.

Hugh Schulze is President and CEO of c|change Inc., a marketing communications company in Chicago, USA. His 25-year career in the communications field has included work in many industries, including healthcare and experience in all media. For the last 10 years, he has served as Communications Consultant for the 'WPA Global Programme to Fight the Stigma and Discrimination because of Schizophrenia' and has spoken at conferences and congresses internationally. He is also Consultant for the WPA Global Child Mental Health Programme.

Reducing the Stigma of Mental Illness

A Report from a Global Programme
of the World Psychiatric Association

Norman Sartorius

and

Hugh Schulze

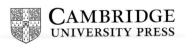

CAMBRIDGE
UNIVERSITY PRESS

CAMBRIDGE UNIVERSITY PRESS
Cambridge, New York, Melbourne, Madrid, Cape Town, Singapore, São Paulo

CAMBRIDGE UNIVERSITY PRESS
The Edinburgh Building, Cambridge CB2 2RU, UK

Published in the United States of America by Cambridge University Press, New York

www.cambridge.org
Information on this title: www.cambridge.org/9780521549431

First published 2005

Printed in the United Kingdom at the University Press, Cambridge

A record for this book is available from the British Library

ISBN-13: 978 0 521 54943 1 paperback
ISBN-10: 0 521 54943 4 paperback

Contents

v

Preface

The Second World War is now becoming a dim memory for all but those who lived it. Among them, those who were not soldiers by profession, civilians caught in the maelstrom of misery, death, terror, starvation and suffering also remember it with particular clarity.

In that war, my mother, a pediatrician, joined the partisans in Yugoslavia and took me along. Although this has been more than half a century ago and I was only 8-year old I still remember the time we spent with the resistance movement with extraordinary clarity: the years immediately before and after have long receded into vague landscapes of time. Among the memories of the war is one of the nasty winter of 1943 when I had an experience that gained in significance over the years.

We had completed many hours of enforced march and had come to a road that we had had to cross: it was well guarded and it was necessary to wait for a period between the enemy patrols to get to the other side. Everyone had to remain absolutely quiet. We held that position for hours waiting for the signal to proceed. It was there that I saw a cortege, a carriage with six white horses, with attendants dressed in eighteenth century costumes and finery pass by on the protected road. It was quite beautiful and I remember how extremely clear it seemed to me. I heard the sound of the hoofs and muted voices of the attendants. The carriage was moving slowly and once it passed another came along. This hallucination lasted for what seemed a long time. When I pointed to the sight and described it to others they looked at me puzzled and ordered me to stop talking about it.

Over the past few decades a number of new findings contributed to our knowledge about schizophrenia. Some of these relate to morphological changes of the brain observable by the increasingly powerful investigative techniques. Others relate to the nature of the schizophrenic experience, to the importance of maintaining the patients' self-esteem for the process of recovery and to the positive role that families can play in helping the patient if properly trained.

And yet, for all the advances that have been made by the neurosciences, by the social and behavioural sciences, by studies of treatment and by public health investigations the mystery of the brain–mind barrier seems as impenetrable as it always was. Jim van Os and others demonstrated that typical symptoms of psychosis appear in people who never consulted a doctor for it with a surprisingly high frequency (Verdoux and Os, 2002): why some of these experiences appear and vanish while others stay or keep coming back and occupy one's mind is still unclear. Why did I see the cortege with white horses when no one else saw it and why did this type of experience never come back even though there were many other situations in which I was exhausted, hungry, sleepy and frightened? And what would have happened to me had I been brought to a hospital, kept there for observation and maybe given some treatment? Could the label of being kept for observation in a mental institution have changed my subsequent schooling, social relationships and working life?

The level of our ignorance is such that it is safe to predict that much more time is necessary before we learn enough about schizophrenia to be able to prevent it. We can however provide care to people who suffer from schizophrenia and know what could enhance the probability that our treatment will be successful and that patients will find their place in society. We know what obstacles stand in the way of recovery and rehabilitation. Among these obstacles undoubtedly the most serious and difficult is the stigmatization of mental illness and of all those in contact with it – the sufferers, their families, the medications used for treatment, the institutions in which treatment is provided, staff in mental health institutions and even the sites on which they are located.

This book is about stigma and ways of fighting it. It reports on what we and the other participants in the WPA Global Programme against Stigma and Discrimination because of Schizophrenia have learned from it. It also contains our thoughts about ways of intensifying the programme and making it an essential part of health services, equivalent in importance to training staff about ways to treat diseases.

We hope that this volume will make readers aware of the nature of stigmatization of mental illness in different cultures and of the consequences of stigma and discrimination for all concerned. We also hope that it will make readers eager to join those who fight these because they are awesome obstacles to progress not only for mental health programmes but also for progress towards the creation of a civil society.

Norman Sartorius
Geneva, Switzerland, 2005

REFERENCE

Verdoux, H. and van Os, J. (2002). Psychotic symptoms in non-clinical populations and the continuum of psychosis. *Schizophrenia Research*, **54**(1–2), 59–65.

Introduction

The stigma attached to mental illness and all that is related to it – patients who suffer from mental disorders, their families, psychiatric institutions, psychotropic medications – is the main obstacle to better mental health care and better quality of life of people who have the illness, of their families, of their communities and of health service staff that deals with psychiatric disorders. It is a basic component of the negative discrimination that people with mental illness experience every day. It blocks access to facilities and options that, in principle at least, have been created to help people impaired by mental illness. Stigma is pernicious and what is worse there are indications that despite advances of psychiatry and medicine stigma continues to grow and has more and more often terrible consequences for patients and families.

The stigma associated with schizophrenia is particularly harsh. A person diagnosed with the illness will be seen by most of those around him or her as dangerous, lazy, incompetent at work, unable to be a family member that fulfills his or her social obligations. Different fears and prejudicial judgments may be in the foreground of stigma in different cultural settings: what is common is that the negative opinion will stay stable even after all the symptoms of the disease have disappeared and after it has been possible to show that the individual concerned can work and fulfill his social roles at least as well as his fellow citizens.

That stigma exists and that it is pernicious is gradually becoming accepted (Link *et al.*, 1992). This growth of awareness is however only rarely accompanied by the commitment or at least willingness to do something about diminishing stigma and its consequences.

The reasons given for inaction by mental health workers (and by others who should be concerned with stigma) are varied. Some say that they are too busy, others that individuals cannot change stigmatization. Still others state that stigma linked to mental illness is not very different from the stigma attached to other illnesses and therefore only a comprehensive programme which is beyond their reach can make sense.

The different voices of stigma and discrimination

During the course of the programme in interviews, in focus groups and more public forums, those living with the illness and their families have described many different ways stigma and discrimination is manifested:

From India: 'My parents support me but we can't tell any of our neighbors. It would hurt my sister's chances of being married.'

From Canada: 'If I apply for the job and tell them I have schizophrenia, I won't be hired. If I don't tell them and they find out, or I suffer a relapse later, I will be fired.'

From Japan: 'Women with an illness like this will be kept at home to do domestic chores, while we men are sent out of the house.'

From the United Kingdom: '[T]he only way I found out the doctors had diagnosed me with schizophrenia was because I managed to read it upside down on my medical notes! No one had told me and finding out that way was very frightening. I felt very alone.'

From the United States: 'The doctors left me waiting in the emergency room, fighting my delusions for six hours; they said other people's problems were more serious than mine.'

The Global Programme of the World Psychiatric Association

In 1996, the World Psychiatric Association undertook a programme to address the stigma and discrimination because of schizophrenia. At a meeting in Geneva, Switzerland, 38 psychiatrists from more than 20 countries and representatives from consumer groups discussed ways to address the barriers to proper treatment, the difficulties with reintegration, and how best to address the human rights of those living with the illness and of their families.

Collectively, the group agreed to three guiding principles for the programme:

- to survey individuals living with the illness and their family members about the experience of stigma and discrimination, and where possible encourage their active participation;
- to encourage the participation of individuals throughout the community whether in health care, government or private enterprise – everyone was welcome;
- to ensure this was a long-term effort, rather than a brief campaign.

To start the programme it was necessary to develop guidelines and manuals. Initially, these would be drafts which would be improved upon in the course of time. To produce those materials the Steering Committee established four other groups:

The *Treatment Committee* was charged with compiling the latest information on the illness and the variety of treatment options available. For the first year, the head of this group was the Italian psychiatrist, Mario Maj. In 1997, Wolfgang Fleishhacker of Austria stepped into that role.

The *Reintegration Committee*, chaired by Julian Leff of the UK, was to examine results of research done on reintegrating individuals back in society.

The *Stigma Committee*, the largest of the four groups, surveyed the manifestations of stigma and discrimination because of schizophrenia in different cultures and countries. Richard Warner from the US directed the efforts of that group.

Finally, while the programme's Steering Committee oversaw the interworking of the groups, the *Review Committee* would review the documents produced by the groups.

After reviewing the evidence and relevant facts, the groups produced a single volume on schizophrenia. The volume was written in the style of an encyclopedia entry, easily readable and based on evidence. The volume was annotated with remarks indicating sections particularly relevant to fighting stigma. This volume was meant to provide a central compendium of the latest scientific information on schizophrenia for the media and programme participants. This volume has been translated into Spanish, Polish, Italian and Japanese. In Spain, it has been published as a book.

The groups next produced a step-by-step guide for implementing an anti-stigma programme. The group understood that most of the implementers of the programme in individual countries would have had little or no experience in addressing public awareness or changing public opinion and wanted to provide guidance on social marketing efforts. That volume was drafted by Dr Sartorius and Dr Hugh Schulze with the help of Dr Warner, and reviewed by the Steering Committee and other experts, such as communication professionals. It is designed to assist psychiatrists and other mental health professionals in assembling a Local Action Group, setting measurable goals and objectives, and identifying key target groups for the programme. The guide includes suggestions on how to hold a press conference, write a press release, and numerous other practical tips. After years of its use, the volume has been further developed through the creation of a Manual with practical suggestions based upon the experiences of the programme and use of the volume.

The steps outlined in that initial volume take Local Action Groups roughly 12 to 18 months to implement – from initial planning meetings to full implementation. Over the years, a number of general principles have emerged that have applied in all countries:

- The programme's goals should be based upon information obtained from patients and their families in the culture in which they live.

- The programme should be directed at particular, defined target groups.
- The programme should be undertaken first in areas in which success is likely in the short term to encourage all participants.
- The programme should include active participants willing to stay with the programme for at least 2 years.
- The Local Action Group should develop a plan of action and invite leading personalities in the country to join the programme's support group.
- The programme will place all of its experience and funding at the disposal of other programmes participating in the global effort, and in turn rely upon their resources when and where necessary.
- When identifying select target groups it is important to have an individual from that particular target group on your team – not only can they provide insights on the best way to address their peers, but recommendations on individuals and groups you may be unaware of.
- For national programs, a group composed of representatives from the different cities or regions is important to ensuring coordination between the groups and amortizing costs overall.
- In general, the more targeted the intervention – in terms of messages and media directed to identifiable individuals or a group – the more effective the effort will be. (We will see examples of this in the Canadian Pilot Study.)

The volume also contained practical suggestions such as the creation of a project log, establishment of regular meeting times and other suggestions for maintaining group cohesion. Examples from both volumes are listed in the appendices of this book.

Since that first meeting, more than 20 countries have undertaken nearly 200 anti-stigma interventions. As we will see, these interventions were directed towards well-defined target groups in an effort to address different parts of the vicious cycles that lead to discrimination and prejudice.

The WPA and Local Action Groups in different countries have published journal articles and reports on the on-going efforts around the world. They have also made presentations at major scientific meetings, conferences and congresses. This book is intended to gather the latest data from all of these efforts and provide insights into how each initiative was developed in a particular country through the cooperation of men and women from a wide variety of backgrounds.

What sets this programme apart from other anti-stigma initiatives is both its international nature – whereby groups in different countries were able to share best practices – and the collaborative nature of the Local Action Groups. Following guidelines set out by the WPA Global Programme and refined in other countries, these groups bring together psychiatrists and other mental health professionals, journalists, politicians, schoolteachers, and perhaps most notably, those living with schizophrenia and their family members as well.

The First International Conference on the Stigma and Discrimination because of Schizophrenia was held in Leipzig, Germany in 2001. In 2002, further findings were presented at the WPA Congress in Yokohama, Japan, a logical consequence of the fact that the Global Programme against Stigma is one of the five Institutional Programmes of the WPA. A Second International Conference was held in Kingston, Ontario in Canada in 2003. It is expected that further conferences dealing with the work against stigma and its consequences will take place and that they will allow an exchange of experience at the same time as an encouragement to those participating in the programme and others that will join them.

Structure of this Book

The opening chapter provides an overview of the challenge and methodologies used to fight stigma and discrimination. The following chapters provide country-specific reports on interventions undertaken following the WPA guidelines. These have been organized more or less chronologically in four phases. Phase I, which involved the first use of Volumes I and II of the programme materials, was undertaken in 1997 in Calgary, Canada. Phase II was an extension of the programme to Spain and Austria. Phase III included other European countries such as Germany. Phase IV was programme implementation in other countries.

Each chapter concludes with a list of articles relevant to the anti-stigma efforts in that country. The final chapter includes a list of recommendations and cautions relevant in undertaking such a programme. In Appendix I, the reader will find Volume I of the programme – a step-by-step guide to planning and implementation. Appendix II contains sample pages from Volume II, which contains information on the diagnosis and treatment of schizophrenia, along with a section devoted to the stigma and discrimination associated with the illness. We have also included the instruments for surveys of knowledge and attitudes that were used in the Calgary Pilot Study in Alberta, Canada.

Additional information is available at the programme web site:
www.openthedoors.com
Those interested in starting a programme against stigma should contact:

Professor Dr Norman Sartorius
14 chemin Colladon
1209 Geneva, Switzerland
Tel: 41 22 788 2331
Fax: 41 22 788 2334
E-mail: mail@normansartorius.com

Please note that those who join the WPA network will be expected to share the data that they obtain in their work with other participating sites and to follow the guidelines of the programme. In turn they will be given access to all of the sites' materials and will be kept informed about the development of the programme.

Participants in the Programme

This programme was developed by experts from many countries, non-government organizations, associations of patients and their families, as well as government representatives.

Steering Committee
Norman Sartorius (Switzerland): Scientific Director
Juan J. López-Ibor (Spain)
Julio Arboleda-Flórez (Canada)
Ahmed Okasha (Egypt): Chairman
Hugh Schulze (United States)
Costas N. Stefanis (Greece)
Narendra N. Wig (India)

Treatment Committee
W. Wolfgang Fleischhacker (Austria): Chairman after 5/97
Juan J. López-Ibor (Spain): Steering Committee Representative
Timothy J. Crow (United Kingdom)
Paramanand Kulhara (India)
Jan Libiger (Czech Republic)
Michael G. Madianos (Greece)
Mario Maj (Italy): Chairman through 5/97
Michael O. Olatawura (Nigeria)

Reintegration Committee
Julian Leff (United Kingdom): Chairman
Costas N. Stefanis (Greece): Steering Committee Representative
Marina Economou (Greece)
Wolfgang Gaebel (Germany)
Ulf Malm (Sweden)
Vincent B. Wankiiri (Uganda)

Stigma Committee

Richard Warner (United States): Chairman
Narendra N. Wig (India): Steering Committee Representative
Anthony W. Clare (Ireland)
Sue Ellen Estroff (United States)
Julio Arboleda Flórez (Canada)
Robert Freedman (United States)
Semyon Gluzman (Ukraine)
Trisha Goddard (Australia)
Driss Moussaoui (Morocco)
Michael Phillips (China)
Everett M. Rogers (United States)
Corinne L. Shefner-Rogers (United States)

Review Committee

Wolfgang Gaebel (Germany): Chairman
Heinz Häfner (Germany): Chairman to 2001
Norman Sartorius (Switzerland): Steering Committee Representative
Istvan Bitter (Hungary)
Giovanni de Girolamo (Italy)
R. Srinivasa Murthy (India)
Ahmed Okasha (Egypt)
Charles Pull (Luxembourg)
Wulf Rössler (Switzerland)
Pedro Ruiz (USA)
Mitsumoto Sato (Japan)
Harold M. Visotsky, deceased (United States)
Greg Wilkinson (United Kingdom)

ex officio Review Committee Members
W. Wolfgang Fleischhacker (Austria)
Julian Leff (United Kingdom)
Richard Warner (United States)

Chairpersons and Advisors of Local Action Groups

Each chapter of this book is dedicated to a different initiative in a different country. At the end of each country report, we will list many of those who have helped make those programmes a success. Here, we wish to acknowledge those heads of sites instrumental in bringing the results to this book. Contact information for individuals and Local Action Groups are given at the end of appropriate chapters. (Like the chapters themselves, the countries are listed in chronological order roughly corresponding to when the initiatives were begun.)

Canada	Julio Arboleda-Flórez and Heather Stuart
Spain	Juan J. López-Ibor and Olga Cuenca
Austria	Werner Schöny and Wolfgang Fleishhacker
Germany	Wolfgang Gaebel and Anja Baumann
Italy	Guiseppe Rossi
Greece	Costas Stefanis and Marina Economou
United States	Richard Warner
Poland	Andrzej Cechnicki and Anna Bielánska
Japan	Mitsumoto Sato
Slovakia	Pĕtr Nawka
Turkey	Alp Üçok
Brazil	Cecilia Villares
Egypt	Tarek Okasha
Morocco	Nadia Kadri and Driss Moussaoui
United Kingdom	Graham Thornicroft and Vanessa Pinfold
Australia	Barbara Hocking and Alan Rosen
Chile	Carlos Caceres Gonzalez
India	R. Srinivasa Murthy and R. Thara
Romania	Raluca Nica

Acknowledgements

This programme would not have been possible without the generous support of many people living with schizophrenia and their families in more than 20 countries around the world, including the family associations that support them. The programme has also been supported by medical and psychiatric institutions, and other agencies many of whom are listed in the appropriate country reports.

We would also like to thank Eli Lilly and Company who have generously supported both the international effort and local initiatives in some countries.

The authors would also like to thank Josette Mamboury in Geneva, Switzerland and Melissa Woods in Chicago, United States for their invaluable assistance in this programme over the years.

Developing the Programme

The World Psychiatric Association (WPA) Global Programme against Stigma and Discrimination because of Schizophrenia was started in 1996 when I became President of the WPA. Initially, we saw it as a policy initiative, not as a specific programme.

My colleagues from the Executive Committee of the WPA (in particular, Professor Juan Jose Lopez-Ibor, then President-Elect of the WPA) and I spoke with possible supporters of an operational arm to the anti-stigmatization policy, including staff of foundations, government agencies, directors of health programmes and representatives of pharmaceutical companies.

While many lauded the initiative, few expressed an interest in joining the effort and even fewer were willing to contribute to a programme in a concrete way. Not so Mr R. Postlethwaite, at the time Vice-President and Director of the Neuroscience Department of the Eli Lilly and Company. He, like others expressed his strong approval of the idea but also sought support from within his company. Dr M. Xilinas, at that time working with Eli Lilly and Company in Geneva, provided invaluable help in the administrative arrangements that followed and WPA soon received a formal confirmation that Eli Lilly would provide some funds to support the initiation of the programme. This enabled us to start the Global Programme and to help its development in the first set of countries that were keen to join the effort.

Thus, in 1996 we brought together a group of people whom we felt could help in the development and implementation of a programme against stigma. The group that met in Geneva included psychiatrists, social scientists, communication experts[1] as well as representatives of family and patient organizations, and government representatives. It reviewed the preliminary plans for the programme, and identified individuals and organizations that could be focal points for its development at country level. The group was invited to address several key, strategic questions including the following:

---

[1] Among them Mr H. Schulze who remained fully involved with the programme throughout and is a co-author of this book.

1 What conceptual framework should the programme adopt?
2 Should the programme be directed to stigma related to a particular disease or to mental illness in general?
3 Who should carry out the programme on a national level?
4 How should the activities composing the programme be selected?
5 What administrative structure should the programme have? Should it be managed by the WPA Executive Committee, outsourced to an agency independent of WPA or carried out by some other arrangement?
6 How long should the programme last?
7 What relationship should be established with other anti-stigma activities underway at the time or initiated at a later date?
8 How should the success of the programme be evaluated?

The guidance received from the group concerning these issues was invaluable in the finalization of the plans for the programme. These will be briefly reviewed, under the headings of the questions presented above.

What conceptual framework should the programme adopt?

Since the early work by Erving Goffman on stigma (Goffman, 1963), many definitions of stigma have been put forward. For the anti-stigma work of the WPA, elements of earlier research and experience were synthesized into an operational model that describes the vicious cycle of mental illness, its stigma and consequences (Sartorius, 2000).

This model has several advantages. First, it acknowledges that 'stigma' should be viewed as one of the important disadvantages created by illness and making it more severe. Second, it stresses that stigma is part of a vicious circle and that it will continue to grow unless the circle is interrupted.

Third, and this is perhaps most important, the cycle identifies access points where interventions might be undertaken and where there is room for action by professionals, social services, hospitals and community agents. The model further shows that there is no one who could not contribute to fighting stigma and its consequences.

The vicious cycle of stigmatization

The model implies that a marker (a visible abnormality) that allows the identification of a person can be loaded with negative contents by association with previous knowledge, information obtained through the press, and memories of things seen in movies or heard in the community.

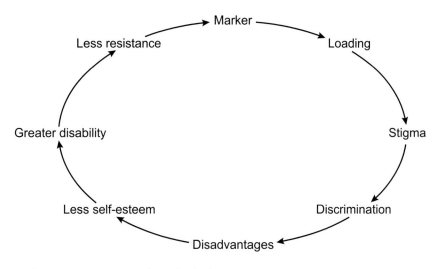

Cycle of stigmatization for the individual.

Once the marker is loaded in this way, it becomes the stigma and anyone who has it will be stigmatized. Stigmatization may lead to negative discrimination which in turn leads to numerous disadvantages in terms of access to care, poor health service, frequent setbacks that can damage self-esteem, and additional stress that might worsen the condition of the consumer, and thus amplify the marker, making it even more likely the person will be identified and stigmatized.

This cyclical model also implies that an intervention at any point might stop that process. Thus, if it proves impossible, for example, to remove stigma it is often possible to focus on removing discrimination by legal and other means.

In other instances, it might become possible to improve treatment and rehabilitation services to a level at which they can offer help to the consumer and the family, and support them in living with the illness. Sometimes it is possible to remove the marker – as in the case with extra-pyramidal symptoms that can appear as side-effects of certain type of medications, but do not appear with other treatments. In some instances, there is enough time and opportunity to educate the community in a manner that will decrease the negative loading of the marker.

A similar cycle can be constructed for families and caregivers. Yet it differs in significant respects.

The shame, guilt and worry that family members can feel adds to stress on the group. This might be just the parent and the child with the illness or encompass a much larger extended family, close friends, coworkers and/or neighbours. The increased stress may reduce the individual's or group's reserves – in terms of emotional and often financial resources, and in terms of time that can be spent with members of the family who are not suffering from the illness. The reduced reserve

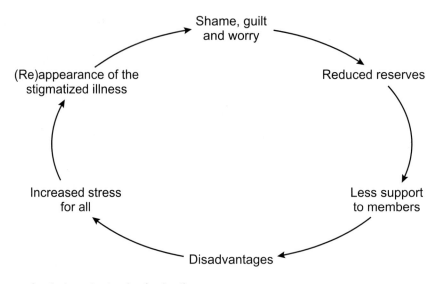

Cycle of stigmatization for the family.

means that family members will have less support in times of need and that as a consequence links among family members can be broken or perhaps even irrevocably severed. This increases the stress for all members of the family or social unit which may lead to a relapse or reappearance of the stigmatized illness. In a manner similar to the circle described for the person with the illness, the family may also lose self-esteem and confidence in itself which makes care more difficult and possibly less effective for those members of the family with the illness.

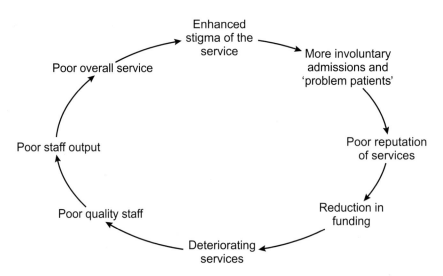

Cycle of stigmatization for mental health services.

Mental health professionals may not be surprised to see this vicious cycle mirrored in the area of mental health services as well.

Family members and those who have developed early symptoms of the schizophrenia, may avoid seeking psychiatric help for a variety of reasons. This may be due to misunderstandings about the illness, its course or the treatments that might be used. But as a number of groups in the WPA programme found in country after country, this may also be due to previous stigmatizing experiences (e.g. dismissive treatment in a hospital emergency room that might include accusations in front of family members of the use of illegal drugs).

Whatever the reasons, by not seeking early treatment, patients may later be admitted involuntarily often with severe forms of acute psychosis. As a consequence, the psychiatric unit or emergency room can come to be seen by other hospital officials and by the population as a holding area for 'problem patients' for whom psychiatric care can do little.[2] The deterioration in reputation of the services in the hospital leads to a reduction of funding.

With a reduction in funding comes a deterioration in services and increasing difficulty to maintain or hire good-quality staff. Poor performance by staff contributes to the overall negative perception of the psychiatric service. As the reputation of the service deteriorates, as word spreads of these poor services, those who may be experiencing early symptoms – or their family members – further stigmatize psychiatric services and delay treatment, perpetuating the vicious cycle.

The impact of the cycles we have described extend beyond those immediately involved at each stage. These cycles reinforce stereotypes, increase cynicism in members of the community, and further diminish hopes of those living with mental illness that things will improve.

These cycles of stigmatization are not isolated from each other. A family that has lost hope and self-esteem will find it more difficult to seek help and realize its right to help. This will not only worsen the situation but also contribute to the perception of weakness of the family and all of its members, and lessen their ability to become active participants, along with the healthcare professionals, in the recovery of the family member with schizophrenia.

These interrelated cycles of stigma and discrimination because of mental illness illustrate specific points for intervention. The next question becomes one of how finely focused the interventions should be.

---

[2] With the current tendency to reduce the number of in-patient facilities, it is often necessary to admit severely disturbed chronic patients with comorbid conditions, both physical and mental (e.g. drug abuse). This further reduces the number of beds available to the service and heightens the threshold for admission for those with early forms of illness who would particularly benefit from appropriate help and treatment.

> ## Cultural differences between industrialized and developing countries
>
> In the 1970's, the World Health Organization (WHO) carried out a major international collaborative study on Schizophrenia (International Pilot Study of Schizophrenia, IPSS and WHO). The study demonstrated that schizophrenia could be found in all nine countries studied (US, UK, India, Colombia, Nigeria, Denmark, Czechoslovakia, USSR and China); that the incidence of schizophrenia did not show much difference among countries, and that the course and outcome of schizophrenia was better in *developing* than the developed countries. Other studies undertaken in the same countries (and some others) confirmed these findings (WHO 1979, Sartorius 1996). The explanation of these findings evaded the investigators: they examined the frequency of stressful events for patients and expressed emotions of family members but the new findings did not help. It might be that the different forms and levels of stigmatization in Third World countries made the difference. It is hoped that a study to explore this hypothesis will be carried out.

Focus on schizophrenia or on mental illness in general?

There are strong arguments for either of these two options. It could be argued that taking all mental illnesses as a target might – if the programme is successful – help incomparably more people than the prevention or removal of stigma concerning a single disease such as schizophrenia. A point in favor of the broad focus could also be that the general public does not make a distinction between mental illnesses and that therefore engaging support of a wide section of the population might be more difficult if a psychiatric label is used in defining the focus of action. Targeting many mental diseases, it was felt, might help to engage a larger number of patient and family organizations. The question of equity also arises if only one disease is selected as a target for action: why should other illnesses not receive the same benefits of a campaign?

The WPA programme decided to take only schizophrenia as a focus for the programme. The arguments for it are numerous and seem to prevail over the reasons for taking all mental diseases as the target. Schizophrenia as a syndrome is a paradigm of mental illness and the general public when asked to describe a mentally ill person invariably lists symptoms such as delusions and hallucinations – hallmarks of schizophrenia – as the defining features of a 'madman'. Stigma related to schizophrenia is more pronounced than the stigma attached, say, to anxiety states or dementia of old age. A success in the prevention or removal of stigma related to schizophrenia would show the way to those fighting to remove the stigma of other mental illness and indeed of other stigmatizing illnesses (e.g. leprosy or syphilis).

The selection of schizophrenia as the central focus of the programme makes the definition of the programme activities less complicated and the evaluation of success easier. Although some non-governmental organizations – for example the World Schizophrenia Fellowship – did excellent work to help people with schizophrenia there was at the time no coordinated international project by a professional or governmental organization that dealt with the disease and could attract the attention of the government and other authorities to the need to support care for people with schizophrenia and their families – arguably the most wretched group among those struck by mental illness.

Who should carry out the programme on country level?

Experience from previous studies and in particular from the international studies on schizophrenia one of us (Norman Sartorius) had coordinated while working at the WHO strongly suggested that the guarantee for a success of a study or other project at country level is not the commitment of the government or of an institution but *the decision of an individual or of a small group of people to carry out the project*. The support of the institutions and governmental agencies is helpful and often necessary but never sufficient. The programme thus expanded to countries in which there was a small group of people willing to lead the action and maintain it over years.

The groups that we sought were to be small. As a rule of thumb, we said, the group should be a size that would allow it go for a meal together in a single car. Such an action group was to ensure support of a larger group of patrons – persons of importance and influence – that could be invited to become members of the Advisory Group for the programme and were likely to be willing to meet at regular intervals (but not too frequently) to receive reports of the action group and to help it by advice, comment and influence to carry out the programme.

How should the activities of the programme be selected?

The advice of the group at the Geneva 1996 meeting was to develop a set of specific plans that would be offered to the action groups in the countries together with an estimate of the time necessary and allowable for the execution of each activity in the plan. This would essentially be what has been described as a collaborative project (Sartorius and Helmchen, 1981). It was felt that this would help to maintain the identity of the programme and facilitate the exchange of experience and evaluation.

As it turned out this advice was neither realistic nor very helpful. Consultations with the potential heads of action groups in the countries and with others involved in similar work indicated that a different strategy was necessary. This new strategy seemed dangerously similar to a plan for confusion as it turned out it became a hallmark of the programme and its most useful feature.

In brief, the strategy of the programme became the reliance on the advice of persons most directly concerned with problems related to stigmatization and discrimination. In each of the sites the first step of the action groups was an exploration of consequences of stigma and discrimination for people with schizophrenia, their families and others who were involved in the provision of care and in the rehabilitation of those disabled by schizophrenia and its consequences. This preliminary exploration usually resulted in a long list of complaints and problems reported by those concerned. The action group then examined the reports and divided them into those that were due to stigma and discrimination, and others that had little to do with them. Among the former group of problems the action group selected targets for action using several criteria: the probability that the problem can be resolved relatively quickly (the more difficult to resolve the less attractive was it for the programme, particularly in the beginning), the likelihood that the problem can be tackled by the action group (with the support of the Advisory Group), the availability of support for work on that problem – either in the form of influence or concrete support of an institution or agency.

The results of proceeding this way were that the programme sites have selected different targets for action and that the speed of their progress varies. This might be seen as a disadvantage, particularly for reporting about the programme and for its evaluation. These shortcomings are however significantly outweighed by the fact that it is easier to find support for the programme that is locally relevant, and that the action group and other participants in the programme knew that they were working on problems that were particularly important for their area. A moral advantage of this way of proceeding was also that action was harmonious with a main objective of the programme – that of contributing to the self-esteem of persons affected by schizophrenia by giving them an opportunity to decide on the course of action and participate in it, thus treating them as equal and making them partners in the programme development.

What administrative structure should the programme have?

The administration of a large-scale programme must be in a single location and the coordinating office has to function continuously from the same place. In view of the fact that the central office of the WPA was traditionally moving to the home site of the Secretary General, the office of the Global Programme against Stigma was separated from the WPA Secretariat and placed in Geneva. A Steering Committee of the programme was created to give its strategic guidance and streamline activities. It was chaired by the President of the WPA and composed of five persons, of whom one was the Scientific Director of the programme. The Office of the programme maintained close collaboration with the Secretariat of the WPA that was also keeping the accounts and ensured auditing. The Steering Committee created four working groups (listed on page xv) dealing with:

1 the distillation of knowledge about schizophrenia and its treatment,
2 the rehabilitation of the patient, and the diminution of stigma and discrimination in the immediate surroundings of the patient,
3 stigma and discrimination in society at large,
4 the review of materials produced by the other three groups.

A web site was created in 1998 to leverage the information already developed and also to provide a global 'brand' – a unified look-and-feel – for the overall effort.

The chairpersons of the action groups in the countries functioned as the parliament of the programme in that they examined, discussed and approved proposals for programme activities reaching across the sites.[3] An instruction guideline was drafted giving a sequence of steps in the programmes at country level. (See Appendix I.) The sequence – for example concerning the formation of the action group, the collection of information, the establishment of the Advisory Group – was recommended for all sites: the timing of the steps as well as the selection of activities at country level was left to the decision of the Local Action Groups and their partners. Annual meetings of all the Heads of sites and biannual meetings of the Steering Committee often together with the Chairpersons of the working groups also served to facilitate the coordination and conduct of the programme.

How long should the programme last?

The Geneva meeting was divided on that question: while some thought that the programme should have the nature of a campaign lasting at the most 2 to 3 years, others felt that the programme should have a longer perspective. The advocates of the former drew attention to the fact that the funding available to the programme were very limited and that planning for a long-term project without a secured source of funding and a strong institutional backing would be an exercise in vain. The advocates of the longer perspectives drew attention to the need for a lasting engagement in all efforts aiming to change attitudes and to the fact that the initiation and conduct of international projects takes a much longer time than activities at a one-country level.

In reality, and to the surprise of many, the programme continued growing and becoming stronger over the years. Now in its tenth year of existence the programme

---

[3] For a listing of members of the Steering Committee, Working groups and Heads of sites, see xxi–xxiii.

still strongly attracts new groups and is expanding its activities. In some of the sites
the tempo diminished, for a variety of reasons – personal, financial and political.
The unavoidable attrition has however been much less serious than feared. The
recognition of the fact that the decrease of stigmatization and discrimination needs
a long time and that short campaigns can bring more disappointment and problems
than no campaign at all also contributed to the credo that a programme against
stigma must be planned to last for a number of years, much longer than other
activities in the field of health.

What relationship should there be with other efforts dealing with problems of stigma and discrimination?

The WPA programme had the advantage that it could examine a variety of efforts
to combat stigma and discrimination because of mental illness in various countries. Some of them were directed against a specific illness, others had a broad
focus. Some dealt with mental illness only and others with increasing tolerance
for those who are different. Most of them were short lasting, some had a solid
backing of an institution or an organization, and others started independently and
worked without much support. Each of these actions against stigma contained
some useful message or experience that could be employed in building the WPA
programme: none however was sufficiently close to it to require fusion or other
arrangements nor was there much competition for funds or other resources with
these programmes. The Geneva meeting therefore recommended that the WPA
programme staff should assemble descriptions of as many programmes against
stigma and discrimination as possible and ensure an exchange of information with
those that were active. Making an effort to include already advanced programmes
under the aegis of the WPA did not seem fair to those who developed their programme – because they might lose some of their visibility – nor useful to the WPA
programme which had to develop its own strategy and tactics being, potentially
the largest and most innovative programme in existence.

How should the programme be evaluated?

The question of evaluation of success attracted much attention during the Geneva
meeting. The usual comparisons of achievements with the objectives seemed
appropriate in some instances but not in others. The essence of the WPA
programme was that it was not a multinational study but an action programme
and a model from which others could learn. The second of these aims imposed the
need for evaluation of the success of each of the component activities so that those
who wanted to learn from the WPA effort could select those of proven usefulness

in another setting. The former objective of being an action programme carried however two other obligations with it: first, that progress should be measured by the extent to which activities against stigma and discrimination became part and parcel of the routine health and mental health programmes; and second that those who have identified problems and difficulties because of stigmatization and discrimination – persons suffering from schizophrenia and their carers – see that some of the difficulties diminish and some of the problems related to stigma that they had vanish.

Snapshots of a dynamic programme

The nature of a Global Programme underway in different countries on different continents is that each report from any one country will be a snapshot of results to date. As this book was being produced, new efforts were underway for establishing Local Action Groups in Zambia, the Czech Republic and Switzerland.

A significant amount of research has been conducted in the last few years on stigma and mental illness by Professor Wülf Rossler and others in Switzerland (Lauber *et al.*, 2001; Nordt *et al.*, 2003; Zogg *et al.*, 2003; Lauber *et al.*, 2004). In 2004, Beate Schulze, whose work with the anti-stigma efforts in Germany, Italy and Slovakia is described later in this book, joined Dr Rossler in Zürich, Switzerland and a Local Action Group has been formed to begin to develop interventions based upon the WPA Global Programme model. These efforts and others are on-going.

The interventions and results presented in this book represent nearly a decade's worth of work in 20 countries. While each Local Action Group developed a programme based upon country- and site-specific challenges of stigma and discrimination, this international approach has allowed us to determine clear patterns and similarities, and provide recommendations for other individuals and groups who seek to fight the stigma and discrimination because of schizophrenia, in particular, or mental illness, in general.

REFERENCES

Goffman, E. (1963). *Stigma: Notes on the Management of Spoiled Identity.* Engelwood Cliffs, Prentice Hall.

Lauber, C., Diebold, H.S. and Rossler, W. (2001). [Attitude of family of psychiatric patients to psychiatric research, especially to early detection of schizophrenic psychoses.] [German]. *Psychiatrische Praxis,* **28**(3), 144–146.

Lauber, C., Nordt, C., Falcato, L. and Rossler, W. (2004). Factors influencing social distance toward people with mental illness. *Community Mental Health Journal,* **40**(3), 265–274.

Nordt, C., Muller, B., Lauber, C. and Rossler, W. (2003). Increased stigma through a former stay in a mental hospital? Results of a public survey in Switzerland. *Psychiatrische Praxis,* **30**(7), 384–388.

Sartorium, N. *et al.* (1996) Long-term follow-up of schizophrenia in 16 countries. [A description of the International Study of Schizophrenia conducted by the World Health Organization.] *Social Psychiatry and Psychiatric Epidemiology,* **31**(5), 249–258.

Sartorius, N. (2000). Breaking the vicious cycle. *Mental Health and Learning Disabilities Care,* **4**(3), 80.

Sartorius, N., Helmchen, H. (1981). Aims and implementation of multicentre studies. *Modern Problems of Pharmacopsychiatry,* 16: 1–8. Basel, München, Paris, New York: Karger.

WHO (1979). *Schizophrenia: An International Follow-up Study.* New York: John Wiley & Sons.

Zogg, H., Lauber, C., Ajdacic-Gross, V. and Rossler, W. (2003). [Expert's and lay attitudes towards retrictions on mentally ill people.] [German]. *Psychiatrische Praxis,* **30**(7), 379–383.

Phase I

Calgary, Alberta, Canada

2

The Canadian Pilot Site

On 16 September 1997, the World Psychiatric Association (WPA) held a press conference during a meeting of the Canadian Psychiatric Association in Calgary, Alberta. The press event was to announce that Calgary would be the pilot site of the global programme to fight stigma and discrimination because of schizophrenia.

Three psychiatrists spoke to journalists about the importance of fighting stigma and discrimination – not only as an issue of social justice but as imperative to effective treatment of schizophrenia. Then, a young woman, by the name of Michelle Miserelli, stepped to the podium and introduced herself as a consumer and a mother who had been invited to speak about the challenges first hand.

'When I first announced that I was pregnant,' she told the attendees, 'my mother's friends asked "When is the abortion going to take place?" That's stigma, a big stigma.' Save for the sound of video cameras and recording equipment the room fell silent. She went on to talk about her 7-year-old daughter. She talked of the challenges of finding a job. 'If I tell an employer I have schizophrenia, I won't get the job. If I don't and the employer finds out later, I could be fired.'

For some of the journalists in attendance, it was the first time they had heard an individual with schizophrenia admit to the illness and describe the discrimination she faced. Working with journalists would remain a key element of the efforts of the Local Action Group in Canada.

Calgary, Alberta

Calgary is located in the Western Canadian province of Alberta. In 1997, its population was roughly 900,000 – most of those are descendents of immigrants from Europe. The rest being immigrant communities from the Asia-Pacific region. Situated east of the Rocky Mountains and west of the badlands and hoodoos of Drumheller Valley, the city was completely transformed when oil was discovered in the region in the 1970s. Within a decade, the town that had been known primarily for its annual rodeo, called the Calgary Stampede, became the Canadian centre for the energy industries and the financial centre of Western Canada.

Calgary was selected as the Pilot Site of the programme for programmatic and pragmatic reasons:

- Canada has well-developed mental health services. Groups in Canada such as the Schizophrenia Society were already involved in combating discrimination. It was thus reasonable to expect that success of the anti-stigma effort would mean that the WPA programme has the potential to make a positive impact even in highly developed countries with well-organized services.
- Professor Julio Arboleda-Flórez, the Local Action Group leader, and his wife, Heather Stuart, were both members of the Stigma Committee and held posts at the University of Calgary. Dr Arboleda-Flórez was Professor and Head of the Forensic Division and Dr Stuart was Associate Professor in the Department of Community Health Services and Epidemiology.
- The educational and healthcare systems were deemed strong. Literacy rates are generally 99% in the urban regions.
- Local consumer and family support systems were also present and strong.
- It was easy to identify a control group to examine whether the programme in areas with fewer health services. A collection of nearby communities to the east in Health Region 5 afforded an excellent opportunity. The town of Drumheller, located in Health Region 5, has a population of 5000.
- Representatives of the Drumheller area and from the provincial capital of Edmonton were also active participants in the Local Action Group. Those from the Drumheller area would help implement the programme in their community; those from Edmonton would prepare the province for expansion of the programme to another major urban centre and facilitate work with the provincial government.
- The city also had a variety of media outlets with some national exposure to reach the general public: more than 30 radio stations, three broadcast television stations, cable television, local and national newspapers, as well as opportunities for billboards and transit cards.

The Canadian Local Action Group first met in June 1997. Over the course of the next 18 months, the group would number 28 members. At any one meeting, however, 14 to 18 members were in attendance.

Professor Arboleda-Flórez assembled individuals from a broad range of areas: two Faculties of Medicine in the Province, academicians associated with the local Day Hospital, officials from the Department of Health of the Government of Alberta and the Alberta Provincial Health Board, as well as Regional Mental Health Service advisors. He also invited a journalist from Calgary's largest circulation newspaper. The involvement of a member of one of the target groups would become an important factor in the success of this and other country interventions. A local representative from Eli Lilly and Company, which provided some funding for the programme, volunteered his time as did all the members of the Local Action Group.

Individuals living with schizophrenia from the Schizophrenia Society of Alberta, the Calgary Clubhouse Society, and the Canadian Mental Health Association participated in the Local Action Group. Representatives from several of these groups were meeting for the first time. As part of a global initiative, groups that had not been actively working together had found common ground, after many years of working separately and sometimes at cross purposes. This would be a dynamic of programmes in other countries as well (e.g. the UK).

The first major task undertaken by the Local Action Group was the development of a survey instrument. The goal was to establish benchmarks for knowledge and attitudes before and after the initial intervention. This research would also serve to shape messages and media selection.

Results from the pre- and post-test results have appeared in several academic papers. One point to stress in the strategic approach to addressing the stigma and discrimination because of schizophrenia was that in Canada a focus was placed on measuring and changing attitudes. In subsequent interventions in other countries, focus shifted to assessing the experiences of those living with schizophrenia and on actions to directly diminish discrimination and its consequences rather than changing attitudes.

A telephone survey was conducted in August 1997 of 600 households in Calgary, and 400 households in the Drumheller region (98% of the homes have telephones). The questionnaire (presented in Appendix III) inquires about an individual's knowledge of the causes of schizophrenia and his or her attitudes toward that individual through questions of social distance. This includes questions such as 'Would you feel afraid to have a conversation with someone who had schizophrenia?'

Eighty percent of those surveyed said that 'schizophrenia did not touch' their lives. Overall, however, the Calgary population appeared knowledgeable about schizophrenia and expressed generally low-perceived stigma, a fact which ultimately may have made the efforts of the group more challenging. The programme began with the bar already set high.

With results of the research tabulated and the official announcement made at the press conference, the group was ready to create a communication plan.

First, the Calgary Local Action Group identified specific target groups. The target groups were: Health Care Professionals (including emergency room personnel, medical students, senior health care policy-makers and general health professionals); Teenagers in grades 9 and 11; Community Change Agents (such as the clergy, business community leaders and journalists); and finally, messages directed to the general public through the mass media.

Among the 20 different countries that have already undertaken the WPA anti-stigma programme, the Calgary group began with one of the largest collection of target groups. While this was in part due to the large size of the group that would develop and the three regions represented (Calgary, Drumheller and Edmonton), as a Pilot Programme they also sought to gather as much experiential data as possible for other groups.

The Local Action Group then split into subgroups to address each different target audience and the various components of that target audience. These subgroups were asked to undertake a 'Zero Budget Exercise' to explore various communication channels for their target audiences that did not require a financial investment, such as the purchase of a mail list or media buy.

At the end of a 4-month process, by December of 1997, the Local Action Group had mapped out specific interventions for each target audience and a timeline for intervention. With this communication plan in place and with specific targets and outcomes identified, individuals of the Local Action Group were then able to approach potential sources for funding.

In March 1998, Beth Evans, a Local Action Group member who also worked with the Provincial Mental Health Advisory Board (PMHAB), was able to secure government funding ($75,000 Canadian). Eli Lilly Canada provided funding for media purchases. In addition to all of the time volunteered by the group members (including travel and meetings), Professors Arboleda-Flórez and Stuart provided meeting rooms and clerical support through the University of Calgary.

The following results are organized relative to the target groups chosen. To better describe the overall effectiveness of these interventions, we will outline the results of the efforts within subgroups.

Health care professionals

Emergency room professionals

The group that took on the task of working with health care professionals included health care professionals and individuals living with schizophrenia. This group conducted surveys of the opinions of patients with schizophrenia, as well as members of the PMHAB and the Alberta Health Authority. Among the findings: while a presentation of policies governing patient rights was formalized in Calgary hospitals, the Drumheller General Hospital had no policy in place at that time for presenting a statement of rights to a patient. For example, none of the hospitals provided a private interview room in the emergency room for psychiatric patients.

The group then submitted the results of this research and five recommendations (the recommendations are listed in the box opposite) to hospital directors and emergency room directors. Members of these subgroups discussed the findings with these individuals and then followed up on the progress of these recommendations.

These recommendations were also submitted to the Canadian Council on Health Services Accreditation. Today, those five recommendations have been integrated into the country's national accreditation process.

The importance of group diversity and consumer input

The health care professionals subgroup was composed of a psychiatrist, members of the Regional and Provincial Mental Health Advisory Boards, and a consumer. The consumer representative reported on the first-hand experiences of other patients who, suffering from acute psychotic episodes, faced stigma upon entering a hospital emergency room (e.g. doctors and nurses often first assumed these individuals were suffering from drug overdoses).

By focusing on this specific point of encounter and stigmatizing behaviour, the group was able to affect one of the greatest changes achieved by the programme, the adoption of five recommendations as part of the national hospital accreditation process:

- That the examination and interview process and space are adequate for safety, security and privacy of patients and staff.
- That there are enough interview rooms available to ensure privacy during interviews in most situations.
- That those interview rooms are located near or with easy access to hospital security personnel.
- That security staff are available in a timely, as needed, basis.
- That a policy is in place for governing the use of restraints.

Medical students, senior health care policy-makers and general health professionals

While the results of the intervention in hospital emergency rooms have been clear and quantifiable, results among the other subgroups of health care professionals were less pronounced but still positive.

Medical students in Edmonton were exposed to an educational intervention that featured an anti-stigma video (developed by Johns Hopkins University). The goal of this intervention was to assess the change in attitudes after approximately 2 h of instruction. There was an increase of 10% in knowledge and attitudes as measured by pre- and post-test results. Work to assess whether an increase of knowledge can be obtained in other ways and whether it is accompanied by changes in attitudes is still being conducted before full integration of this educational component into the medical school curriculum.

Two interventions were aimed at senior health care policy-makers. First, a presentation of the efforts in Calgary and Drumheller was made to the PMHAB, which resulted in additional funding to continue the anti-stigma work.

The second involved presentations and efforts to achieve at least one policy change in each of the following areas: housing, employment, income and the availability of proper drug treatment. As these were not more thoroughly defined (e.g. what kind of change in employment?) and because numerous groups lobby both the Regional and Provincial Advisory Boards for such changes, the impact of the Local Action Group is difficult to assess. For example, while availability of proper drug treatment has been achieved, whether this was the result of private company lobbying or the Local Action Group's efforts is difficult to determine.

For general health professionals, members of the Calgary Schizophrenia Society had written and produced a play which is performed by individuals living with the schizophrenia. The drama is called '*Starry, Starry Night*' after the song by Don McLean about the life of Vincent Van Gogh. All of the roles – doctor, nurse,

---

Starry, Starry Night

In the course of the WPA global programme, a number of different Local Action Groups have undertaken theatrical productions to describe for audiences the experience of schizophrenia as well as the stigma and discrimination experienced. Future chapters on Poland and Germany will feature other such examples.

Here are some of the observations from Fay Herrick, Director of the Schizophrenia Society of Calgary, on the experience of the '*Starry, Starry Night*' production in Calgary and Health Region 5:

'The first performance was huge because we did not know if we could do it. The cast members were all very nervous and I was really afraid of the scene where David is crushed by the voices. We had only rehearsed that scene once and every member of the cast was in tears.

Two other performances stand out in my mind. On October 22, 1999 we performed the play for 480 people who were attending the Schizophrenia Conference in Edmonton. Our players were rewarded with a loud standing ovation that lasted a very long time. This performance brought tremendous recognition in Alberta for our programme and for our members.

The other very important performance was the performance in Kingston, Ontario at the international conference in October 2003. This invitation to perform came at a time when our group really needed a lift. To be invited to perform our play for people from different countries has given all of our members a sense that our efforts are worthwhile.'

mother, girlfriend and the main character, David – are played by individuals living with the illness. Players read from a script which reduces the stress associated with memorizing dialogue. The production follows David through the course of dealing with his hallucinations (a scene in which all the players surround David as the voices oppressing him), to speaking to the doctor and dealing with side effects of his medication, to conflicts with his girlfriend and family.

Working with the Schizophrenia Society, the Local Action Group was able to have the play presented in eight Calgary hospitals and one in the Drumheller region. Six years after those performances, 'Starry, Starry Night' is still performed in hospitals around the province. It has not been possible to quantify the effect (e.g. changes in attitudes) of the play in these settings. What is certain is that the performers report that the participation in the play has given them much in terms of self-esteem and friendship with other players.

The players also travelled to Kingston, Ontario and presented the play at the *Second Annual Conference on the Stigma and Discrimination because of Schizophrenia* in October 2003. Attendees assessed it as one of the highlights of the conference, highly praised by all.

Teenagers: students in grades 9 and 11

The Local Action Group further developed a successful intervention with junior and senior high school students in Calgary and Drumheller. This target audience was chosen *a priori* (i.e. not because this group was identified on the basis of a survey or qualitative study) bearing in mind that first symptoms of schizophrenia are often experienced in one's teen years and that in other studies it could be shown that changing knowledge and attitudes of children and adolescents had an effect on their parents and the community as a whole.

The group's efforts were built upon an existing programme of the Calgary Schizophrenia Society called the 'Partnership Programme'. This programme is a 60- to 90-min presentation given by both a consumer and a family member. Students are thus given two perspectives on the illness, on its course and treatment and the stigma and discrimination associated with it.

A good deal of data now exists on the stigma-reducing benefits of first-hand interactions with those suffering from mental illness. Witnessing these presentations first hand, it is obvious that students are fully engaged and remain concerned with what they heard. While certain descriptions of delusions may cause a titter to ripple through the classroom (one young man related with self-deprecating humour how he had come to believe the wife of pop star Paul McCartney was in love with him and was trying desperately to get in touch with him), students usually have open, frank and respectful dialogues with presenters on issues ranging from sexuality and the effects of medications to feelings of loneliness (for both the consumer and family member) and social policy (such as issues of institutionalized discrimination in housing or health care).

However, getting into schools was at first not an easy proposition. 'When I first began calling schools to discuss an educational programme,' Fay Herrick, Director of the Calgary Schizophrenia Society, recalls, 'people would listen politely but when they heard the word "schizophrenia" they couldn't get off the phone fast enough. It took time but gradually, as the good news about the presentation spread, it became a little easier.'

Affiliation with the WPA global programme helped open a few more doors. The number of speaker's bureau presentations in Calgary increased from 10 to 15 per month. The number of participating junior and senior high schools increased from 31 to 44. While there had been no presentations by the Partnership Programme in the Drumheller area up to that point, through the efforts of Local Action Group members Monica Flexhaug, Maureen Drake and Marian Ewing, by fall of 1998, the Partnership Programme was making five presentations a month. By January 1999, twelve schools in the Drumheller area were actively participating.

These presentations achieved significant changes in knowledge and attitudes.

In Calgary:

- The proportion of high school students expressing no social distance increased from 16% to 22%.
- The proportion expressing the highest degree of social distance fell from 13% to 8%.
- The median knowledge score increased from 7 to 8 on a 9-point scale.
- The proportion of students achieving a perfect score increased from 11% to 19%.

In the Drumheller area:

- The proportion of high school students expressing no social distance increased from 13% to 32%.
- The proportion expressing the highest degree of social distance fell from 19% to 4%.
- The median knowledge score increased from 7 to 8 on a 9-point scale.
- The proportion of students achieving a perfect score increased from 8% to 31%.

The figures are indications that change did occur and that it went in the right direction.

The Teens Talking 2 Teens Competition

In order to actively involve teenagers in the anti-stigma effort, the Local Action Group held a competition for junior and senior high school students. Students were challenged to develop media materials that would inform other teens about schizophrenia and the effects of social stigma on those living with the illness.

Competitions were held in the Spring and Fall of 1998. (See the sidebar for more information on the messages and communication tools used.) Students wrote poetry, shot videotaped vignettes, painted posters and created a web site. During the Fall of 1998, 35 students from Calgary high schools submitted entries. Teens in Health Region 5 entered 25 creative presentations.

The mayor of Drumheller and a representative from the Calgary Regional Health Authority attended the awards presentation in the Drumheller area health region

Getting the message right

The importance of the involvement of people living with the illness in selecting target audiences and developing messages is important. Similarly, it is important to have a member of a target group in the Local Action Group (a journalist when educating journalists; a judge when dealing with the judiciary) and to test messages with, if possible, a representative sample of the target audience.

The development of posters for the 'Teens Talking 2 Teens Competition' provides one notable example. Several different graphical designers put together a dozen rough concepts for the poster. When these were presented to the Local Action Group, the adults – all over the age of 25 – voted for the poster shown on the left below. The cartoon characters were seen as non-threatening, warm and human. The dialogue balloons were thought to be an engaging way to detail facts about schizophrenia. On the other hand, the poster at the right, featuring the human brain, was deemed 'too edgy, too scary' and that the depiction of multiple brains might reinforce misunderstandings of 'split personality'.

The group agreed, however, to show the posters to a number of teenagers. The teens overwhelmingly chose the poster on the right. The bright colours and distressed type matched graphics they were familiar with from MTV and video games.

Not only was the artwork adopted for the high school poster, but it was also used as the front cover of the Teacher's Manual, a special manual that the Calgary group developed for distribution to teachers. When adults in the group saw the popularity of the graphical, a request was made to change the contest copy at the bottom of the poster and use the poster for describing efforts of the WPA global programme at meeting of the Canadian Psychiatric Association.

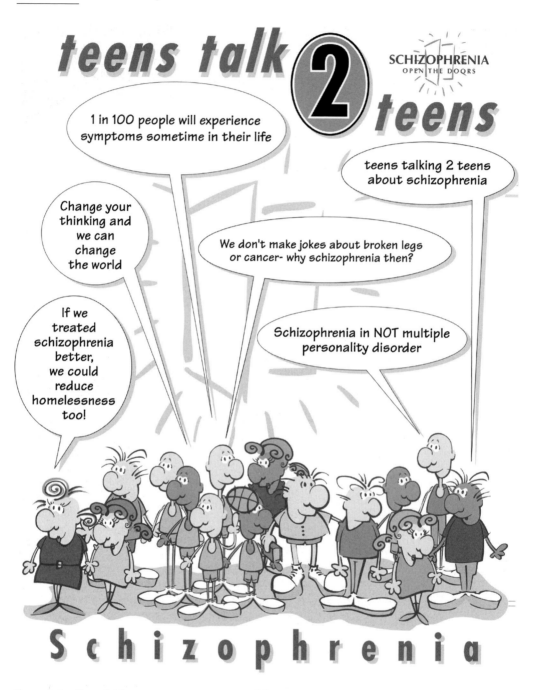

Figure 2.1   Two of 12 poster concepts presented for a competition in Calgary junior and senior high schools. The poster on this page was the one chosen by adults on the Local Action Group. The poster on the next page was chosen by teenagers in the target audience

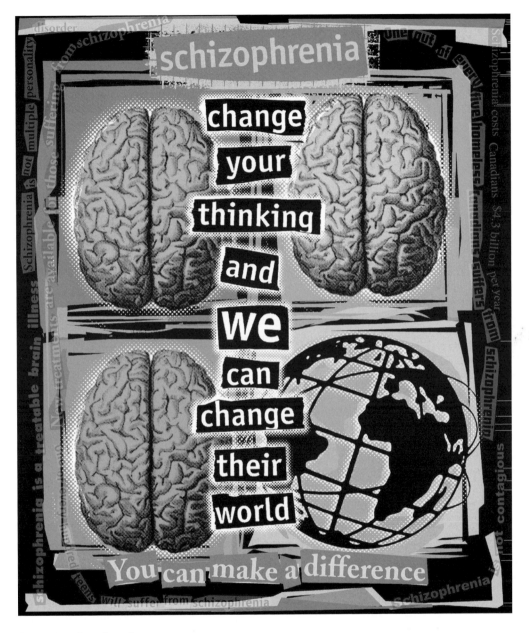

Figure 2.1   (*Continued*)

in January 1999. Winners of the contest received plaques and cash awards of $100 and $50 (for first place and honourable mentions, respectively).

Six years later, the contest continues in Calgary junior and senior high schools. Winners are awarded their prizes during Mental Health Awareness Week, when public figures, such as the mayor participate in the formal ceremony.

The '*Teens Talking 2 Teens Competition*' was also adopted by the Local Action Group in Boulder, Colorado. As we will see, winners from this competition have had their artwork featured on transit cards, placed inexpensively in public buses along routes to and from area schools as well as on the web site of the Boulder Community Mental Health web site.

Community Change Agents and opinion leaders

Everett Rogers, in his book *Diffusion of Innovations*, defines Change Agents as:

an individual who influences clients' innovation-decisions in a direction deemed desirable by a change agency… One of the main roles of a change agent is to facilitate the flow of innovations from a change agency to an audience of clients.

The Calgary Local Action Group sought to target change agents in three groups: clergy, business community leaders and journalists.

For *clergy* in Calgary and Drumheller areas, the goals were well-defined: Partnership Programme presentations to 20 church congregations and youth groups; presentations by ten youth groups to their congregations; placement of phone numbers for assistance in 30 church bulletins along with a 250-word description of the stigma campaign; and presentations given to minister groups. The outcome objectives were: to have 10% of congregation members and youth group respondents report a significant improvement in knowledge and attitudes; for ministers of these congregations to know the principle symptoms of schizophrenia and to know where to refer someone with possible schizophrenia or other mental illnesses.

Unfortunately, the results were mixed at best. Presentations were given to five congregations, six ministers' groups in Calgary and one large ministers' meeting in Drumheller. Pre- and post-testing was inconsistent and ultimately measurement of how well ministers understood and recalled the information that was presented is unclear.

Results for *business community leaders* were disappointing as well. Goals were set to target both chief executives and human resource departments to make presentations in their companies and solicit contributions for the anti-stigma effort. While presentations were made at two Chamber of Commerce meetings and human resource directors of 15 corporations were contacted, it proved impossible to recruit a business leader to the Local Action Group, and little or no real measurable progress was made.

The third target, *journalists*, achieved significant results. Forty press kits were mailed to journalists in the region and personal contact was established with 30 of these journalists in Calgary and seven in the Drumheller area. The goal of the group was to increase positive news coverage by 10% between calendar 1997 and 1998.

When the final results were assessed, the actual outcome was an increase of 35% in the number of positive news stories in the local paper with the largest circulation, the *Calgary Herald*. A comparison was made in two consecutive 8-month periods following the campaign, compared to the 8 months prior to the campaign. The average length of those positive stories increased 16%.

All of this happened in spite of two high-profile headline stories with negative content associated with schizophrenia: the Unabomber trial in the United States and a story in the Canadian press of a man who pushed a commuter from a subway platform in Toronto. During the two 8-month periods following the start of the programme, stories with negative news coverage associated with schizophrenia increased 44%.

What accounted for the marked difference between these three groups of opinion leaders and change agents? The most important reason was the presence of a representative from the target audience on the Local Action Group. Bob Bragg, a journalist from the *Calgary Herald*, worked closely as part of the group, helping to shape messages and make contact with other journalists. In a series of columns that immediately followed the press conference in September 1997, he related the first-person stories of Michelle Miserelli and other individuals living with the illness and worked to dispel some of the myths and misunderstandings that surround schizophrenia. In a later chapter, we will see how a journalist had a different kind of impact on efforts in Saõ Paulo, Brazil.

Neither clergy nor local business leaders were represented in the planning group. Despite the best efforts of those in the Community Change Agent subgroup, access to these individuals was limited.

Dr Richard Warner, who would start a programme in Boulder, Colorado a year later, was able to apply lessons learned in Calgary and achieved good results with the local business leaders. The results of that intervention are presented in Chapter 8.

Who *is* the general public?

In the early planning stages of any Local Action Group, it is not uncommon for a discussion to turn to an anti-stigma programme complete with an all-out media barrage on television – 30-s commercials produced by directors who have won the Palme D'Or, speaking engagements with talk show celebrities, news segments on Fuji Television, CNN and Al-Jazeera. Certainly the dream of broad reach and social impact is part of even the smallest Local Action Group effort. The efforts of the Greek Programme in hosting a major concert event with the international diva,

Nana Mouskouri, would never have occurred if the group had not aimed high. But the realities of financial and human resource limitations often rein in such dreams.

As we will see in the case of Austria, taking a public awareness programme to television can achieve some tangible results. However, before engaging in such activities it is important to keep one key point of social marketing in mind: there is no such thing as the 'general public'.

Advertisers of consumer products have long understood that the more targeted the message and media choice, the more likely they are to achieve their goals. Hence the choice of some commercials (e.g. beer and sports utility vehicles) placed during football games and others (e.g. financial services and cars) during news programmes. While this may seem at first to be self-evident, the discipline of staying 'on message' and the practice of pre-testing with an intended audience has only been applied in the last few decades to everything from the promotion of movies to political campaigns.

In Germany, the Local Action Group involved with the WPA anti-stigma pro-gramme used focus groups, small group discussions conducted with a moderator. Focus groups have been used extensively in consumer advertising for many years. The goal is to more effectively gather qualitative research and explore how products and messages might be refined.

Having said all of that, the question becomes: is the use of mass media (e.g. tele-vision, radio, billboards) a cost-effective expenditure for social marketing efforts? With the WPA anti-stigma programme, the results have varied from country to country. In the case of Canada, where 60-s messages were broadcast on three radio stations, the group was effective in creating Awareness but changes in Attitudes were disappointing. (The cost of a 60-s spot in radio during drive time was a fraction of the cost of a 30-s spot in television's prime time – both in terms of production and media placement.)

The radio spot featured the voice of Dr Ruth Dickson (chair of the programme from September 1998 to December 1999) and one of three individuals living with schizophrenia. In industry terms, the 60-s recording was a 'doughnut', a standard opening and close to bookend the spot, and an open centre in which alternate messages could be placed. This structure allowed the placement of alternate mes-sages to reduce the cost of production, and also increased the recognition of the overall series. Dr Dickson recorded an opening and closing message on stigma and discrimination against those with schizophrenia, along with a phone number that listeners could call for more information. At the centre of the 'doughnut' was one of the three recorded first-person accounts of those living with schizophrenia.

The radio spots were played on three local stations, CKIK, CJAY and CKRY, for 2 weeks in the morning and afternoon as commuters were on their way to and from work in the last 2 weeks of January and all of February 1999. These three stations were chosen because their formats skewed to younger adult audiences (which research showed was less stigmatizing and include teenagers who had seen Partnership presentations in their high schools and young adults of an age more likely to develop early symptoms of schizophrenia). The music formats of these three stations also differed (e.g. CKIK featured 'adult contemporary' pop and rock and CKRY is a country music station), allowing the group to reach more listeners.

Additional funding allowed the commercials to be run again later in the year for Mental Health Awareness week. However, post-testing needed to be conducted after the first placement in January/February for data to be collected and submitted to the Steering Committee.

Anecdotally, for members of the Local Action Group, the results were 'overwhelmingly positive'. In the first 2 weeks, the radio spots generated dozens of phone calls. Members reported colleagues in hospitals and in health agencies relating that they had heard the messages. Dr Ruth Dickson reported that a year after the last spot had been aired patients or family members entering the clinic still mentioned they had heard her on the radio.

Post-testing in March indicated that between a quarter and one-third of those surveyed (28%) recalled hearing the messages. Extrapolated to the population of Calgary, roughly a quarter of a million people heard, and remembered, the messages.

And yet, research on attitudes showed no statistically significant shift in public attitudes. It should be noted, however, that in addition to research being conducted after only the initial flight of messages, as we saw earlier, during the course of the Pilot Programme negative news coverage by journalists increased 44%.

In future chapters, we will deal with the use of mass media by Local Action Groups in other countries.

Conclusion

The number of target audiences (and the groups within those categories) chosen in Canada exceed those of nearly all other Local Action Groups involved in the WPA global anti-stigma campaign. By engaging in more activities, this group was able to learn lessons which would prove instructive to later efforts (e.g. the importance of a member of a target audience within the Local Action Group).

The effort in junior and senior high schools achieved significant, measurable change in knowledge and attitudes in both urban and rural settings. As of this writing, presentations by the Partnership Programme continue in these schools, as does the '*Teens Talking 2 Teens Competition.*' (Artwork of the winning efforts of students have been featured in a calendar distributed during Mental Health Awareness Week.)

Significant, national change in policy was achieved when focus was placed on emergency room admission procedures. While results with medical students and general health professionals have been less dramatic, the existence of on-going informational presentations within these influential groups is clearly a positive outcome.

Among opinion leaders and change agents, efforts directed toward journalists yielded more positive press coverage. Much work is still needed to eliminate misconceptions and misunderstanding (such as the routine use of 'schizophrenic' for inconsistent behaviour from everything from sports teams to politicians) perpetuated in newspaper headlines and on television.

Finally, in the use of mass media for broader reach in the city and outlying areas, messages by the Local Action Group were heard – and recalled – by an estimated quarter of a million people. While generating community awareness is one way to build public support that will move politicians and other civic leaders, more study will be required to see how these messages affect attitudes in the long term.

All of these changes were achieved in the 2 years after Michelle Miserelli spoke to the press. More continues to be done by individuals who were involved in the Local Action Group as well as by Fay Herrick and her group with the Calgary Schizophrenia Society.

Before all of the Canadian results were tabulated, two other initiatives of the WPA's global anti-stigma effort had begun. The next two chapters will examine the efforts and results in Spain and Austria.

For more information on the Global Programme in Canada, please contact

- Julio Arboleda-Florez (Advisor)
  Department of Psychiatry, Faculty of Medicine, Queen's University
  Kingston, Ontario, Canada K7L 3L6
  Phone: (+1-613) 544 3400
  Fax: (+1-613) 547 1501
  E-mail: jearflo@aol.com
- Fay Herrick
  Schizophrenia Society of Alberta, Calgary Chapter
  #700-2310 2nd Street SW
  Calgary, AB, Canada T2S 3C4
  Phone: (+1-403) 264 5161
  Fax: (+1-403) 269 1727
  E-mail: ssacc_advocacy@telus.net

• Heather Stuart
Department of Community Health and Epidemiology,
Abramsky Hall, Queen's University
Kingston, Ontario, Canada K7L 3N6
Phone: (+1-613) 533 2901
Fax: (+1-613) 533 6686
E-mail: hh11@post.queensu.ca

BIBLIOGRAPHY – CANADA

Arboleda-Florez, J. (1998). Mental illness and violence: an epidemiological appraisal of the evidence. *Canadian Journal of Psychiatry – Revue Canadienne de Psychiatrie*, **43**(10), 989–996.

Arboleda-Flórez, J. (2002). What causes stigma? *World Psychiatry*, **16**(1), 1.

Arboleda-Florez, J. (2003a). Considerations on the stigma of mental illness. *Canadian Journal of Psychiatry – Revue Canadienne de Psychiatrie*, **48**(10), 645–650.

Arboleda-Florez, J. (2003b). Life is like an onion. *Academic Psychiatry*, **27**(3), 223–224.

Arboleda-Florez, J., Holley, H. and Crisanti, A. (1998). Understanding causal paths between mental illness and violence. *Social Psychiatry & Psychiatric Epidemiology*, **33**(Suppl. 1): S38–46.

Holley, H. (1998). Quality of life measurement in mental health. Introduction and overview of workshop findings. *Canadian Journal of Community Mental Health*, **3**(Suppl.), 9-20, 9-21.

Rogers Everett M. (2003). *Diffusion of Innovations*, 5th edn. Free Press, New York, NY.

Stuart, H. and Arboleda-Florez, J. (2001a). A public health perspective on violent offenses among persons with mental illness. *Psychiatric Services*, **52**(5), 654–659.

Stuart, H. and Arboleda-Florez, J. (2001b). Community attitudes toward people with schizophrenia. *Canadian Journal of Psychiatry – Revue Canadienne de Psychiatrie*, **46**(3), 245–252.

Thompson, A.H., Stuart, H., Bland, R.C., Arboleda-Florez, J., Warner, R., Dickson, R.A., Sartorius, N., Lopez-Ibor, J.J., Stefanis, C.N., Wig, N.N. and WPA, World Psychiatric Association (2002). Attitudes about schizophrenia from the pilot site of the WPA worldwide campaign against the stigma of schizophrenia. *Social Psychiatry & Psychiatric Epidemiology*, **37**(10), 475–482.

Phase II

3

Spain

In 1997, a celebration was held in Madrid to mark the thirtieth anniversary of the Clinica Juan Jose López-Ibor. The clinic's founder, J.J. López-Ibor had achieved considerable notoriety in the 1950s for a publication on human sexuality. A decade earlier, he achieved a different kind of celebrity when he and other Spanish intellectuals were placed under house arrest by Francisco Franco. In 1964, 3 years prior to the opening of his clinic in Madrid, he was voted the third president of the World Psychiatric Association (WPA).

That evening, his son Juan J. López-Ibor Aliño, addressed the gathering of psychiatrists and dignitaries. Professor López-Ibor Aliño and several of his siblings had followed their father into psychiatry and 2 years later, in 1999, he would step into his father's former position as president of the WPA.

Also speaking that evening was a representative from the Vatican in Rome, Dr Joaquin Navarro-Valls. Statistics place the number of baptized Catholics in Spain somewhere between 96% and 99% of the population. While the presence of such a high-ranking member of the Catholic Church was one reason for the attentiveness of the audience, another was the subject of the talk: social stigma and the depersonalization of the individual as major impediments to treatment. Navarro-Valls spoke to those assembled at the clinic of the need to see the face of God in the faces of those living with mental illness.

That same year, the Local Action Group, assembled by Professor J.J. López-Ibor Aliño conducted a comprehensive survey among the general public, and more specifically, among patients, family members and mental health professionals. The survey was conducted by a professional research firm and the findings caused the group to take a very different approach to addressing stigma and discrimination from the Canadian pilot test.

Research with the general public revealed that only 17% had heard or read something about schizophrenia in the previous 6 months. A surprising 83% reported that they knew nothing about the illness. One-third of the remaining group said they did not know the causes of schizophrenia and 44% said there was no cure.

While knowledge and awareness were low, so too was the public's reported stigma and discrimination. Eighty per cent of those surveyed, for example, would be in favour of having a treatment centre for schizophrenia in their neighbourhood.

Yet, those living with schizophrenia, their family members and health care workers all reported high levels of stigma and discrimination. Forty-two per cent of the families said that the individual could not marry; 52% said they could not have children and nearly one-third (29%) said they could not have a relationship with a member of the opposite sex.

In contrast, no psychiatrist questioned, denied the ability of those living with schizrenia to have a relationship with a member of the opposite sex. Only 2% said they should not marry and 5%, that they should not have children.

When the individuals themselves were asked, 8% believed they could not have a boyfriend or girlfriend. Ten per cent said they believed they could not marry.

On the question of schooling and study, 95% of the psychiatrists responded that those living with schizophrenia could study. Yet 33% of the people living with the illness reported that they had a limited capacity. The rates were even higher for family members: 69% believed the individual could not study.

Although a majority of those living with the illness believed they could recover, 78% of family members said this was not possible. Equally disturbing, 60% of psychiatrists consider it unlikely a patient will improve. For this reason, those living with the illness are treated as highly incapacitated, chronic patients needing a great deal of assistance.

Given these statistics, it is not surprising to learn that the majority of people with schizophrenia feel rejected because of the illness and reported feeling rejected by their psychiatrist.

Psychiatrists in turn felt rejected by the families of those with the illness (52%) because families see no improvement and do not accept the diagnosis. They also feel rejection by the patients. Fully 30% of psychiatrists surveyed felt rejected by other health care professionals because they 'provide few solutions' and that psychiatry itself was 'not very useful.'

A survey conducted by the Madrid Association of Friends and Families of those with Schizophrenia confirmed the social impact of such fatalistic thinking: 62% of those living with the illness engage in no type of productive activity. Eighty per cent live with their families, but do not provide any financial support. While family support appears to be higher than in many industrialized countries, the illness disrupts the relationship with the family and others in the community in a significant manner.

Working from the inside out

Based upon these findings, the Local Action Group in Madrid developed what it called an 'inside-out' strategy for addressing the stigma of schizophrenia. That is, they would begin the anti-stigma interventions working with those closest to the illness. Given the disparity of knowledge and attitudes among patients, their family members and psychiatrists, the group developed an educational program to address the myths and misunderstandings of the illness, and the stigma that can arise from this lack of knowledge. With each target audience, the circle would be expanded outward to increase knowledge among other health professionals (including the staffs of hospital emergency rooms, a focus of the Canadian intervention), then to legal, labour and educational decision-makers.

The Madrid approach may be instructive for countries where, stigma and discrimination in the general population is relatively low, compared to that reported among members of the immediate family or health care professionals who are in direct contact with the individual. The concern of the Local Action Group was that with such little public knowledge about the illness, its course and outcome, a public awareness campaign might actually increase stigma.

The Local Action Group was, however, able to receive funding for a public relations (PR) initiative to disseminate information about schizophrenia, and the advances in treatment to the scientific press and the news media. Before addressing that effort, we should examine the coalition of both groups in the public and private sectors who supported the program.

Before initiating any intervention, the planning group in Madrid secured support from the Ministry of Health and Human Services (Ministerio de Sanidad y Consumo), the Ministry of Work and Social Policy (Ministerio de Trabajo y Asuntos Sociales) and the National Drug Policy Plan (Plan Nacional Sobre Drogas). In addition the Federation of Patients and Family Member Associations (FEAFES), the Association of Health Journalists (ANIS), and the pharmaceutical company, Eli Lilly and Company, leant their support. After initial implementation in Greater Madrid, the group would refine the programme based upon feedback and take it nationally into all 14 autonomous regions of Spain.

One of the first actions taken with the funds raised was to translate Volumes I and II of the programme materials into Spanish. Volume II would later be edited and printed in book form, given the title: *Qué es y cómo se trata la esquizofrenia y cómo combater el stigma*. This book would serve as the support text for the educational programme for psychiatrists, individuals living with the illness and family members. After an initial publication and distribution of 1000 free copies, the book was offered for sale.

Interventions for individuals living with schizophrenia and their families

The Technical Secretariat of the Local Action Group worked in collaboration with consumer and family organizations to develop informational presentations. In Madrid, 78 psychiatrists participated in a programme entitled 'Schizophrenia Without Stigma' during which individuals living with the illness and members of their family were given a choice of 49 different informational presentations. Today, several thousand Spaniards living with schizophrenia and their family members have participated in educational programs akin to that programme.

In the 3 years, from 1999 to 2002, more than 178 psychiatrists participated in lectures, conferences, and other media events with persons living with schizophrenia and family members throughout all regions of Spain. The goal of these presentations was to develop a more open dialogue among all the parties in this inner-most circle of influence with the illness. Psychiatrists have been better able to share the latest information on schizophrenia and new treatment regimens, while individuals living with schizophrenia and their families have been better able to educate psychiatrists on the lived experience of schizophrenia and the various manifestations of stigma and discrimination they encounter, often during treatment.

Health care institutions

Professor J.J. López-Ibor Aliño and the programme's technical secretary coordinated presentations for the 'Open the Doors' anti-stigma programme in two state and six regional institutions during 2000. Such presentations, detailing the stigma and discrimination faced by those living with schizophrenia, were also given to officials in the Health and Consumption Ministry (General Secretary of Sanitary Cooperation) and in the Work and Social Affairs Ministry (General Secretary of Social Affairs).

The group also made presentations on the local level to the Consejería de Sanidad (Local Health Authorities) in Madrid, Castilla y León, Baleares and Comunidad Valencia. In addition to the authorities who participated in the programme in Andalusia and Santa Cruz de Tenerife, presentations were given in 14 other Spanish cities: Barcelona, Badajoz, Burgos, Cádiz, Logroño, Lugo, Murcia, Oviedo, Palma de mallorca, Pamplona, Segovia, Valencia, Valladolid and Zaragoza.

In follow-up research conducted in 14 of the 17 autonomous regions in Spain, the Local Action Group found a decrease in the shame expressed by families regarding a son, daughter or sibling's schizophrenia. The 'inside-out' strategy appears to have been effective in addressing the stigma and discrimination expressed in the closest circles of influence.

An approach to the public

Unlike the other pilot sites, Canada and Austria, the group in Spain decided to work with a PR firm rather than an advertising or marketing agency. As discussed earlier, one of the reasons for this is that given the low awareness and knowledge of schizophrenia, its treatment and outcome, the group feared social marketing might generate more questions and raise more fears than it answered or eased.

In the private sector, most companies and corporations with significant marketing budgets pursue *both* advertising and PR. For non-profit organizations with limited budgets working with either communications channel can be a financial hardship. However, each has its relative advantages.

Advertising allows a group, the greatest control over message content and placement. This control comes at a cost of both time and money insofar as placement of a single 30-s television spot on prime time television in the United States costs thousands, sometimes tens or hundreds of thousands, of dollars. But most countries have broadcast guidelines that mandate networks broadcast a certain number of hours of public service advertising for free or discounted rates. (Even this option can prove problematic if television stations relegate these commercials to late in the evening when airtime is less expensive and less of a financial loss.) Depending on the magazine, newspaper, or radio station, other advertising media can be far less expensive and allow for longer messages.

PR firms have established relationships with members of the press. These firms can be effective in pitching stories to editors or broadcasters. These stories can range from brief interviews with professional psychiatrists in conjunction with a new story or event (e.g. providing a balanced, medical perspective if an individual with mental illness is involved in a crime) to entire news segments or informational programs. Perhaps more important than any single story are relationships PR firms can establish with reporters and editors who may be seeking intelligent (and sometimes photogenic) sources for comment.

As with media purchases of advertising, PR access is more or less directly proportional with a group's financial investment. One other trade-off to consider is that messages disseminated through PR channels gain editorial credibility by being reviewed and published (or broadcast) by a reputable news organization. However, the trade-off for this editorial credibility compared to advertising is some loss of control and repeatability. The most brilliant interview can be bumped from the evening news by a breaking story. Similarly, interviews may be fresh news today when they are relevant to a local conference or event, but by week's end it may be old news.[1]

---

[1] We should mention one other recent media development in this area which may be useful for some anti-stigma programmes. Video News Releases (VNRs) have become packaged ways in which pre-scripted

Working with one of Spain's leading PR firms, Llorente y Cuenca, the group was able to place more than 184 journal and newspaper articles, during the first 3 years of the programme. In 2003, roughly two dozen more articles appeared.

Broadcast media coverage, including interviews and news segments referring to the stigma and discrimination because of schizophrenia totalled 1 h and 30 min of television coverage and 2 h of radio time. The firm has estimated that an equivalent amount of air time (purchased as advertising) would have cost 212,715,905 pesetas (1,376,700 USD). Combining the reach of both the print and broadcast exposure, the group calculates it reached an accumulated audience of 91 million, adding up to multiple exposures in a country with a population of 34 million people over the age of 15.

The anti-stigma programme itself, 'Open the Doors', has been featured in medical journals, and radio and television programmes. Working with Llorente y Cuenca, the group has held press conferences in 13 cities across Spain.

The group also arranged media events during the release of the film *A Beautiful Mind*. Like other groups in other countries, the Spanish Local Action Group scheduled meetings and symposia to coincide with the release of this award-winning film, based on the life of Nobel Prize winner John Nash. Public events, such as these afford an opportunity to encourage further discussion of issues and answer questions raised in such films.

Results

The 'inside-out' strategy of working with those closest to the illness was effective in reducing the shame reported by family members with a son, daughter or sibling living with schizophrenia. On a national level, the Local Action Group was especially effective in recruiting the support of psychiatrists nationwide to implement the educational programme – a data point other programmes may wish to consider, whether the community of change agents be psychiatrists, journalists or some other profession.

Results from the PR effort, however, revealed an interesting and challenging paradox. In research conducted in 14 of the 17 Spanish regions, knowledge and attitudes about schizophrenia increased. In 2000, 26% of those surveyed said that an individual with schizophrenia could have a normal job. In 2001, that number rose to 48%.

However, when asked in 2000 if they would allow a day centre in their neighbourhood, 81% said they would. In 2001, that number fell to 76%.

---

video footage can be provided to news outlets. Based on the same principle as a press release for the print media, a VNR allows an organization to prepare its own news segment which might then be edited by a television or radio station. With greater production control over the creation of the VNR, the group can hone interviews and other footage as necessary, complete with a voice over narrator. For better or worse, corporations and political groups have begun to use this communication channel more often to better polish their messages.

The increase in reported social distance is cause for further investigation and for consideration by other groups where knowledge about schizophrenia is low.

In March 2004, Professor López-Ibor and Dr Olga Cuenca met Fernando Lamata, the new General Secretary of Health (Secretario General de Sanidad) to discuss government involvement in fighting the stigma and discrimination because of mental illness. In June 2004, initial planning was begun for a national programme to address issues of stigma and discrimination.

For more information on the Global Programme in Spain, please contact

- Olga Cuenca (Coordinator)
  J.A. Llorente and O. Cuenca
  Hermanos Bécquer, 4-6^a 28006 Madrid, Spain
  Phone: (+34-91) 563 77 22
  Fax: (+34-91) 563 24 66
  E-mail: ocuenca@llorenteycuenca.com
- Juan J. López-Ibor Aliño (Advisor)
  Clinica López-Ibor
  C./Nueva Zelanda, 44, E-28035 Madrid, Spain
  Phone: (+34-91) 373 73 61
  Fax: (+34-91) 316 27 49
  E-mail: jli@lopez-ibor.com

BIBLIOGRAPHY – SPAIN

Garcia, J. and Vazquez-Barquero, J. (1999). [Deinstitutionalization and psychiatric reform in Spain.] [Spanish] Desinstitucionalizacion y reforma psiquiatrica en Espana. *Actas Espanolas de Psiquiatria*, **27**(5), 281–291.

Giron, M. and Gomez-Beneyto, M. (2004). Relationship between family attitudes and social functioning in schizophrenia: a nine-month follow-up prospective study in Spain. *Journal of Nervous and Mental Disease*, **192**(6), 414–420.

Jacobsson, L. (2002). The roots of stigmatization. *World Psychiatry*, **16**(1), 1.

López -Ibor Alino, J.J. (2001). [Fight against schizophrenia stigma.] [Spanish] La lucha contra el estigma de la esquizofrenia. *Anales de la Real Academia Nacional de Medicina*, **118**(2), 295–316; discussion 317.

López-Ibor Jr, J.J. (2002). The power of stigma. *World Psychiatry*, **16**(1), 1.

Montero, I., Asencio, A.P., Ruiz, I. and Hernandez, I. (1999). Family interventions in schizophrenia: an analysis of non-adherence. *Acta Psychiatrica Scandinavica*, **100**(2), 136–141.

Ochoa, S., Haro, J.M., Autonell, J., Pendas, A., Teba, F., Marquez, M. and NEDES Group. (2003). Met and unmet needs of schizophrenia patients in a Spanish sample. *Schizophrenia Bulletin*, **29**(2), 201–210.

4

Austria

In the midst of frenetic commercials selling soaps, jeans and politicians, the television screen is held in seeming freeze frame: a close-up of a telephone answering machine. An incoming call activates the tape recorder and we watch the wheels spin. But for the duration of this spot, no voice speaks. The phone is not hung up. The mysterious caller appears to be unable to say what he or she wanted to say. At the machine switches off, the titles appear:

Schizophrenie hat viele Geschicte
Sprachlosigkeit ist eines davon

'Schizophrenia has many faces – speechlessness is just one.' This statement is followed by a toll-free number, which the viewer can call for help or more information.

This television spot, winner of a bronze award in the Austrian Commercial Competition, was run on national television in September and October 2000. At the same time, posters in buses and transit stations presented other 'faces of schizophrenia'.

Geography undoubtedly played a role in the Austrian Local Action Group's choice of television as a medium to communicate their message – as it did in the choice for Austria to be the first of the three pilot site countries to start the programme as a national effort. Austria is one-sixth the size of Spain. The province of Alberta where the Canadian programme began in Calgary is larger than Spain and Austria combined ($661,848\,\text{km}^2$). The greater metropolitan region of Madrid is home to a population that is now more than half the total population of Austria. In the country of $83,858\,\text{km}^2$, the Austrian Broadcast Corporation (ORF) reaches more than 4.5 million people daily, roughly 55% of the population.

Professor Wolfgang Fleischhacker, who had served as chair of the Treatment Committee of the World Psychiatric Association (WPA) anti-stigma programme, worked with Dr Werner Schoeny and others to establish working groups in Salzburg, Linz and Vienna. These three urban centres each included members from three national organizations: Österreichisch Gesellschaft für Neurologie and

Psychologie, Österreichische Schizophreniegesellschaft and Pro Mente Sana. The latter two were patient and family organizations. The involvement of both professionals and individuals living with schizophrenia became a hallmark of most WPA efforts. In Austria, the central, organizing action group was composed of two individuals living with schizophrenia, one family member, four psychiatrists, two other mental health professionals, a business leader and a public relations specialist.

Establishing a benchmark

Unlike Canada and Spain which conducted research and then defined target audiences based upon that research, the group in Austria identified four target audiences and then conducted knowledge and attitude surveys among these groups. The target audiences chosen were: public schools, general mental health assistance services, psychiatric institutions and journalists.

Using the instrument developed in Canada, they interviewed roughly 2000 adults with representative samples from each target audience. While each of the groups expressed varying levels of stigma, journalists demonstrated significantly higher levels of stigma to the illness.

While 80% of the doctors surveyed identified genetics as the main cause, 70% of the general population listed stress as a probable cause and 60% thought that head trauma could cause schizophrenia. A surprising 84% of the general public said they were not interested in hearing more about schizophrenia, indicating a high social distance.

Targeting journalists

Based upon the findings, the Austrian group developed an approach designed to simultaneously use the media to disseminate information and change the knowledge and attitudes of print and broadcast journalists. Working with the Austrian Society of Psychiatry and Psychotherapy, they approached the country's largest newspaper, *Kronenzeitung*. The newspaper agreed to run a weekly page covering mental health issues.

In addition to this regular column, the group pursued an extensive public relations campaign with other newspapers, magazines and the broadcast media. From 1999 to 2002, articles appeared in *Neue Zeit, Die Furche, Salzburger Nachrichten, Tiroler Tagezeitung, Medical Tribune* and *Der Standard*.

Overall, more than 100 articles and news reports appeared in both the print and broadcast media. Articles also appeared in scientific and medical journals, such as *Neuropsychiatrie, Jatros Neurologie u. Psychiatrie, Medical Tribune* and *Ärtzwoche*.

Brochures and press kits dispelling popular myths associated with schizophrenia were distributed to the press. More than 75,000 folders, booklets and newsletters have been distributed to the general public as well.

Educating high school students

Like the Canadian pilot programme, the Austrian group decided to target high school students. In part they chose these teenagers because the first symptoms of schizophrenia commonly occur during the mid- to late-teen years. However, the group also wanted to address myths and misunderstandings early in the classroom setting. In this way, they hoped to avoid the development and entrenchment of stigma and discrimination.

Between 1999 and 2002, more than 130 presentations and educational work-shops were conducted in high schools across the country. By developing a teaching curriculum that could be used in health or science courses at the high school level, the Austrian programme was able to establish regular, on-going presentations in many schools across the country. In 2004, the group then initiated a Campaign for Prevention and Reduction of Suicides – another urgent mental health crisis for this age group in many countries.

As noted earlier, unlike other initiatives that may approach such programmes as short-term 'campaigns', the WPA emphasizes long-term commitment of groups. In this way, educational initiatives that are undertaken in order to fight the stigma and discrimination because of schizophrenia can be both updated with new information and broadened to include such topics as teenage suicide or drug abuse.

Broadening the audience

The Austrian initiative chose to use mass media to reach a wider national audience. Working with an advertising agency, the group created a 30-s television commercial and a shorter 15-s version. Airtime was purchased and the spots were run 32 times in September and October 2000. They were also shown in movie theatres.

The broadcast messages reached 46% of the total television viewing audience (8.1 million viewers) in September and 59% (14.6 million viewers) in October. To coincide with the broadcast of these messages and reinforce them, posters and transit cards were placed on buses and other public transportation.

Four months later, 14% of those surveyed remembered seeing the television spots. More than 500 calls were placed to the telephone number advertising more information about schizophrenia and the anti-stigma effort itself.

Mental health services

As the pilot sites in both Canada and Spain found, individuals living with schizophrenia often identify mental health professionals among the sources of stigma and discrimination. The Canadian programme recommended guidelines for dealing with acute cases in emergency rooms. The Spanish initiative fostered greater communication of information between mental health professionals and the consumer.

In several provinces in Austria, small discussion groups were established for people working in the health and social services. After an initial informational presentation – by psychiatrists and individuals living with the illness – the group engaged in conversation about issues they faced concerning the stigma and discrimination associated with schizophrenia. This participatory approach engaged the attendees in something more than a didactic lecture of information and also allowed them to voice their own frustrations or concerns.

In 2003–2004, the focus of these efforts with those involved in mental health services was expanded to include vocational needs of those living with schizophrenia. Working with the Ministry of Labour, the group is hoping to support those living with schizophrenia already in the workforce with regular intervention and treatment.

Conclusion

While a follow-up national survey still needs to be undertaken to determine if the stigma and discrimination because of schizophrenia have been lowered, numbers do indicate that the message was received by millions of Austrians. The results described above were also published in the scientific journal *Neuropsychiatria*. The group continues its efforts, building on its earlier successes and currently looking for ways to fight institutional discrimination through the legal system.

For more information on the Global Programme in Austria, please contact

- Wolfgang Fleischhacker (Advisor)
  Department of Psychiatry, Innsbruck University Clinics
  Anichstrasse 35, A-6020 Innsbruck, Austria
  Phone: (+43-512) 504 3669
  Fax: (+43-512) 504 5267
  E-mail: wolfgang.fleischhacker@uibk.ac.at

- Fritz Schleicher
  Pro Mente Upper Austria
  Figulystrasse 32, A-4020 Linz, Austria
  Phone: (+43-732) 65 13 55
  E-mail: schleicherf@promenteooe.at
- Werner Schöny (Coordinator)
  Österreichischer Nervenärzte und Psychiater
  Wagner-Jauregg-Krankenhaus, A-4020 Linz, Austria
  Phone: (+43-732) 65 61 03
  Fax: (+43-732) 65 13 21
  E-mail: werner.schoeny@gespag.at

BIBLIOGRAPHY – AUSTRIA

Angermeyer, M.C., Liebelt, P. and Matschinger, H. (2001). [Distress in parents of patients suffering from schizophrenia of affective disorders.] [German] Befindlichkeitsstorungen der Eltern von Patienten mit schizophrenen oder affektiven Storungen. *Psychotherapie, Psychosomatik, Medizinische Psychologie*, **51**(6), 255–260.

Freidl, M., Lang, T. and Scherer, M. (2003). How psychiatric patients perceive the public's stereotype of mental illness. *Social Psychiatry and Psychiatric Epidemiology*, **38**(5), 269–275.

Gutierrez-Lobos, K. and Holzinger, A. (2000). [Mentally ill and dangerous? Attitudes of female journalists and medical students.] [German] Psychisch krank und gefahrlich? Einstellungen von JournalistInnen und MedizinstudentInnen. *Psychiatrische Praxis*, **27**(7), 336–339.

Holzinger, A., Angermeyer, M.C. and Matschinger, H. (1998). [What do you associate with the word schizophrenia? A study of the social representation of schizophrenia.] [German] Was fallt Ihnen zum Wort Schizophrenie ein? Eine Untersuchung zur sozialen Reprasentation der Schizophrenie. *Psychiatrische Praxis*, **25**(1), 9–13.

Merl, H. and Schöny, W. (1983). [The psychiatrist's basic attitude in the treatment of acute psychoses.] Die Grundhaltung des Psychiaters bei der Akutbehandlung von Psychosen. *Wiener Medizinische Wochenschrift*, **133**(12), 311–313.

Schöny, W. (1998). [Schizophrenia – an illness and its treatment reflected in public attitude.] Schizophrenie – eine Erkrankung und ihre Behandlung im Bild der Offentlichkeit. *Wiener Medizinische Wochenschrift*, **148**(11–12), 284–288.

Phase III

5

Germany

In 2002, the movie, *A Beautiful Mind*, John Nash won the Academy Award for the Best Film and Ron Howard won for the Best Director. The movie followed the life of mathematician John Nash from his days as an undergraduate at Princeton when he first developed symptoms of schizophrenia to his Nobel speech in Stockholm.

When the film was released in Germany, another film was receiving a great deal of attention though its international distribution would be far more limited. *Das Weiße Rauschen* (The White Noise) is the story of a Lukas, a 21-year-old college student who develops schizophrenia. The film won the Max Ophüls Newcomer Prize at the Saarbrücken Film Festival. When word spread of the film at the Berlin Film Festival, the single screening – put on for distributors and the press – was standing room only. Exhibitors had to set up a second screening to accommodate those who could not attend the first screening.

Despite the similar subjects of the films – two first-person perspectives on the thoughts, delusions and hallucinations of a person living with schizophrenia – the presentations were dramatically different. *A Beautiful Mind* ends with the central character receiving the Nobel Prize, while *Das Weiße Rauschen* ends more enigmatically with the protagonist standing alone a beach, listening to the roar of the ocean.

How do such powerful depictions of the inner life of those living with schizophrenia alter public stigma and discrimination? Might the frightening and emotional portrayals instill more fear and social distance? Or does a realistic presentation of the experience (at least as realistic as the presentation of an interior experience can be) allow the viewers to better empathize with an individual living with schizophrenia? As we will see later, these were just two of many questions that have been investigated by the different regional groups who have participated in the National Programme in Germany.

Like the Austrian programme, the effort in Germany was undertaken as a national effort with multiple centres – but that's where the similarities end. While German geography (Germany being ten times as large as Austria) made this national approach more challenging in terms of coordination among seven centres, the differences were in many ways more notable than their similarities.

In 1999, the Federal Ministry of Education and Research founded the German Research Network on Schizophrenia (GRNS). This network is one of 17 medical networks created to integrate the work of leading research institutions and qualified routine care facilities. Düsseldorf is the coordinating centre for GRNS. The network includes multi-centre treatment studies, biological and genetic research projects and general topics such as health care economy and training. High priority is given to public education. Professor Dr Wolfgang Gaebel, in his multiple roles as speaker of the GRNS, chairman of the Review Committee of the World Psychiatric Association (WPA) programme and head of the coordinating centre of the German 'Open the Doors' projects, worked with the Steering Committee to develop a close working relationship with the German Research Network.

For that reason, in addition to the awareness-raising efforts of the GRNS, the network has actively promoted the 'Open the Doors' anti-stigma efforts throughout Germany. Through the general public relation activities of the GRNS Head Office, roughly 200 press reports have been released since the network was established. Network members have been involved in nearly 40 radio and television programmes.

A German 'Open the Doors Society' was founded in the year 2000. It involves seven different centres in six different cities and a number of different on-site directors. Professor Gaebel is chairman of the society. The centres include:

- **Düsseldorf** (Coordinating centre). Professor Dr Wolfgang Gaebel, Programme Director; Anja Esther Baumann, MA, Programme Coordinator; H. Zäske, Scientific Co-worker.
- **Leipzig**. Professor Dr Mathias Angermeyer, Programme Director; Dr Manuela Richter-Werling, Journalist, Coordinator.
- **Munich Ludwig-Maximillan University**. Professor Dr Hans-Jürgen Möller, Programme Director; Petra Decker, MA, Programme Coordinator.
- **Munich Technical University**. Dr Werner Kissling, Programme Director; Dr Kerstin Wundsam, Programme Coordinator.
- **Hamburg**. Professor Dr Dieter Naber, Programme Director.
- **Kiel**. Professor Dr Aldenhoff, Programme Director.
- **Itzehoe**. Dr Arno Deister, Programme Director.

Given the number of different centres and the challenge of a national initiative, the WPA enlisted the assistance of four advisors as well: Professor Dr Norman Sartorius, Geneva; Professor Dr Wulf Rössler, Zurich; Professor Dr Heinz Häfner, Mannheim; and the President of the German Society of Psychiatry, Psychotherapy and Nervous Diseases.

Each Programme Director then assembled a Local Action Group consisting of: individuals living with schizophrenia, relatives, journalists, health professionals, politicians, opinion leaders and representatives from relevant target groups. Each group operated independently, assessing needs in a particular community and appropriate responses. All groups then reported their findings back to the coordinating centre in Düsseldorf. These research results are being collected and analysed for presentation in 2005/2006.

For that reason, we will report the efforts of each centre separately. Although some anecdotal results can be reported from individual interventions, the larger report has yet to be written on the effects of this initiative nationwide.

Düsseldorf

In a coordinated effort with other centres of the German Research Network, the centre in Düsseldorf conducted a survey of knowledge and attitudes in: Düsseldorf, Munich, Köln, Bonn, Berlin and Essen. Following this survey, the centres in Düsseldorf and Munich conducted an anti-stigma intervention. The groups in Köln and Bonn conducted an awareness programme on schizophrenia, its treatment and outcomes. Berlin and Essen were the control sites.

A pair of other surveys were conducted. One of the general public, the second a quality of life survey of those living with schizophrenia.

Using an instrument based upon the Perceived Stigma Questionnaire (Link, 1989) and the Alberta Pilot Site Questionnaire, each centre surveyed 1175 members of the general public via telephone.

More than 80% of those sampled stated that more positive media reports, more occasions for personal contact with mentally ill people and more public information about mental illnesses would be useful possibilities to improve the public acceptance of mentally ill patients. Eighty per cent of those surveyed thought that patients suffering from schizophrenia suffer from a 'split personality'. The post-survey with the same interviewees has been conducted in summer 2004, the assessment of the data is currently underway.

The second survey was a quality-of-life survey conducted with 109 inpatients at the Department of Psychiatry and Psychotherapy. The survey was based upon: the Stigma and Discrimination Survey (Wahl, 1999), Lancashire Quality of Life Profile (Priebe and Kaiser, 1999), Global Assessment of Functioning Scale (Endicott, 1976).

People living with schizophrenia reported that most of the discriminating situations they faced were at the workplace. Colleagues or employers were rated as supportive, but this group is also rated as the highest discrimination source.

The national group decided that results of both surveys demonstrated the need for additional information and training activities. The Local Action Group decided to concentrate efforts on reducing the social distance to people with schizophrenia. Activities would be designed to both improve knowledge about schizophrenia and contact with mentally ill people.

Interventions undertaken since 2000

The Local Action Group identified three target groups for interventions: the general public, schoolchildren and journalists. Public awareness and education programmes took a number of forms, including art exhibitions 'Psyche and Art' and 'Ex neuron'. There were also public readings done by patients and actors called 'Wenn die Seele überläuft' ('When the mind (or Soul) overflows'). A theatre event called '4.48 Psychosis' and a benefit concert called 'Katja Riemann: Favourites' also increased the awareness of anti-stigma activities and the problem of stigma and discrimination because of schizophrenia in Germany.

Specific educational lectures and seminars were held at grammar schools and institutes for adult education. To address the target group of journalists, the Local Action Group continues to hold workshops with journalists and work with the media.

A joint research project was conducted by the World Health Organization (WHO) teams in Nürnberg, Germany; and Skopje, Macedonia (working with Drs Richter and Niklewski). The team conducted attitude surveys with the general public in Macedonia and Germany. Results from these surveys were then compared and analysed relative to differences in the health care systems in both countries. Based on these results, the team developed intervention strategies for anti-stigma work in Macedonia. These will focus on interventions with psychiatric hospital staff workers and law enforcement officers.

The first 'Anti-stigma Prize' in Germany

In June 2003, at a countrywide journalism workshop in Düsseldorf, the Open the Doors Society awarded the first Anti-stigma Prize. This has been instituted as an annual award. In 2004, the prize of 6000 Euros was awarded in cooperation with the German Society for Psychiatry, Psychotherapy and Nervous Diseases.

Anti-stigma Training Modules

Based upon the data collected from research and interventions to date, educational modules are being developed and evaluated. These 'Anti-stigma Training Modules' have two components: methodological information about the development, and implementation and evaluation of anti-stigma interventions with particular target groups.

Informational material produced for the special needs of target groups (e.g. 'On Causes of Schizophrenia' and 'On Treatment of Schizophrenia').

These modules will allow individuals and institutions to develop their own anti-stigma interventions to target groups they specify (e.g. journalists, law enforcement officers, schoolchildren psychiatric hospital ward staff and the general public). All of these efforts would be conducted in cooperation with the national 'Open the Doors Society'.

Competence Centre for Destigmatization of People with Schizophrenia

A Competence Centre for the Destigmatization of People with Schizophrenia (CCDPS) will be established under the umbrella of the GRNS in Düsseldorf. This group will provide advice on the implementation and evaluation of modules for a modest fee. These services will include: 'Train-the-Trainers' seminars, evaluation services, and continued updating and further development of the modules, thus contributing to the long-term support and maintenance of the GRNS activities.

Hamburg

The Local Action Group in Hamburg chose high school teachers and students as their target audience. In 1998, they founded the society 'Irre Menschlich' composed of professionals and individuals living with schizophrenia. Their mission was to coordinate education within schools.

In 2003, 20 schools with 35 classes (from 5th grade to 12th grade) were visited, each by a team of one professional and one consumer (a patient or family member). During the first year, the project concentrated on psychoses. In addition to schizophrenia, bipolar disorders, eating disorders, cannabis abuse and borderline disorder were also topics of increasing attention. At each of these educational sessions, participants were given a media package with age specific materials about mental illness, stigma and discrimination.

More specialized courses were also offered in cooperation with the Hamburg Institute for Advanced Training of Schoolteachers.

In an effort to determine the kinds of messages being communicated to school children regarding mental illness, the group conducted an analysis of German books for children and young adults.

Since 1999, an 'Open Door Day' has been organized each year, again focussing on information for schools and the general public. About 3000 pupils and 2500 adults are reached annually.

One pilot project concentrated on personnel managers of medium- and big-sized companies in Hamburg, establishing contacts and inviting them to informational events. This project received major attention; 50 companies are already involved. The two most recent projects are the information of local journalists (of print media and of television) and the support of a stage production written and directed by a former psychiatric patient.

Itzehoe-Steinburg and Kiel

The Local Action Groups in Itzehoe and Kiel joined forces in their efforts to involve community leaders in an existing consumer organization: 'Verein zur Förderung der Integration psychisch Kranker und Behinderter im Kreis Steinburg e.V.' (Society to Support the Social Integration of Mentally Ill and Disabled People in Steinburg County).

An informational campaign was undertaken in this rural region, enlisting area residents in the support of mental health initiatives. In addition, booths were set up at community meetings, discussing health topics and upcoming events showing support and solidary for those with mental illness.

Leipzig

Like both Hamburg and Itzehoe-Steinburg and Kiel, the Leipzig group worked closely with a consumer group. They founded the society 'Irrsinnig Menschlich e.V.' which focuses on public relations in the field of mental health and psychiatry. Its aim is to counteract stereotypes about schizophrenia and other mental illnesses and prejudice towards those suffering from them, by informing people about mental illness and treatment opportunities. It also facilitates greater communication and contact between people with schizophrenia, family members, social scientists, journalists and local politicians. During the course of this programme, they hired a journalist to write press releases for the press as necessary (e.g. to describe activities of the group itself or to correct misreporting by the media).

The projects and activities of the association were developed on the basis of the results of a focus group study assessing the concrete stigmatization experiences of people with schizophrenia and their families.

Focus groups

Focus groups have been used as a qualitative research tool for many years in consumer marketing. Only recently has this technique been applied to the social sciences. Focus groups have been used successfully in countries such as Germany, Brazil and Japan despite cultural difference. Discussions involve 8–12 participants and are guided by a facilitator. Participants discuss a limited number of issues in order to identify a range of opinions and ideas for specific groups.

In the case of anti-stigma interventions, focus groups of those living with schizophrenia or their family members enable Local Action Groups to better understand the challenges of those who directly experience stigma and discrimination.

More important perhaps than simply providing insights, focus groups also:

- empower people living with schizophrenia and family members by acknowledging their expert role and soliciting their assistance in defining effective interventions;
- help identify and recruit interested and qualified individuals for task groups;
- involve members from all relevant groups in programme development and thus help sustain ongoing support throughout the programme;
- help balance the interests of programme planners with the perceived needs of the intended beneficiaries of the programme.

In the final analysis, focus groups produce a rich body of data expressed in participants' own words. In Leipzig, Dr Matthias Angermeyer and Beate Schulze made significant progress in developing more finely honed methodological tools for using focus groups and realizing the benefits listed above.

Interventions based upon Focus Group results: secondary school students

Students, ages 14 to 18, were invited to participate in a creative programme entitled: 'Crazy? So What!' Students were placed in teams with individuals living with schizophrenia to develop a creative project of the groups' choosing – a photo exhibition, a collection of texts or series of paintings. In 2002, 21 schools from Leipzig, Halle and Borna participated in the programme.

Participants in the 'Crazy? So what!' project were given a social-distance questionnaire prior to and after the intervention. Control groups not taking part in the project days are also questioned – to control for other possible influence on attitudes towards schizophrenia during the same period.

In general, research from these programmes found:

- adults are more prejudiced than children and adolescents;
- students' attitudes towards people with schizophrenia improved through the course of the project;
- negative ideas about people with schizophrenia have been reduced during the course of the programme; and
- there is more clarity about the meaning of the word 'schizophrenia' following the course.

Adult education

The Leipzig group also developed an adult education course. The series of evening courses and discussions on mental illness is taught jointly by mental health professionals, people suffering from a mental illness and family members in cooperation with the Leipzig Adult Education Centre. Enrollment in these courses has steadily increased since they were first started in 2002.

Media

Through 'Irrsinnig Menschlich e.V.', the Local Action Group has produced anti-stigma messages in virtually every medium, for example, television reports such as the report 'I Am Schizophrenic, but Not Crazy,' which was awarded the 'Schizophrenie und Stigma' prize for journalism in 2001.

One of the programmes that received a great deal of media attention is a TV documentary film, *The Boss is the Patient*. The film focuses on one of the members of the international anti-stigma movement, Dr Petr Nawka, who has been instrumental in establishing the programme in Slovakia. The film was developed in collaboration with the Slovakian anti-stigma initiative.

This same partnership between Leipzig and the Local Action Group in Slovakia has been responsible for *Media Cell Michalovce – Against the Images in the Head*, a film workshop in Michalovce. The workshop included people with schizophrenia and media professionals from Slovakia and Germany, and was held in July and August of 2002. Eight women and men, diagnosed with schizophrenia, from Slovakia and Germany worked as a team with four media representatives. The media project is a model for future workshops designed to mitigate social conflict between those in the media and those who are often marginalized or excluded from the media process. The film developed in this workshop has been shown to audiences in Slovakia, Germany and other countries at international festivals and showings. A companion book documents the workshop and the working relationship of people living with schizophrenia and media professionals as part of Media Cell Michalovce.

Munich

Two anti-stigma efforts have been undertaken in Munich. The first is through the Ludwig-Maximillian University (LMU). The second involves the Munich Technical University (TU). The LMU centre is part of the German Research Network and both work in close partnership on anti-stigma events such as regional press workshops.

The LMU group organizes events for the general public such as monthly lectures and readings with well-known authors, art exhibitions, cinema shows that include panel discussion and poster actions such as 'Artists Against Stigma'. At many of these activities surveys are conducted, measuring the knowledge and attitudes of the relevant target groups.

Those involved in anti-stigma work at the TU are working in cooperation with 'BASTA' (Bavarian Anti-Stigma-Action). This effort focuses on:

1 educational work in schools;
2 education of law enforcement officials for dealing with the mentally ill in stressful situations;
3 the development of art and cultural projects.

BASTA has also founded 'SANE,' an Internet-based, 'stigma-busting' network designed to fight discriminating advertisements. SANE works with direct mail campaigns to the originators of discriminating publications (e.g. advertisements, TV series, movies and press reports).

The Impact of Cinema

Ron Howard's film, *A Beautiful Mind*, can arguably be called a Hollywood blockbuster. Although it contains no car chases or exploding spaceships, the film earned $170,742,341 at the US box office alone. Based upon the life of Nobel Prize winner, John F. Nash, the movie also won four Academy Awards.

In late 2001, *Das Weiße Rauschen* (*The White Noise*) by director Hans Weingartner played at several German film festivals and won several awards. The director, Hans Weingartner, shot the film to give the viewer some sense of the experience of schizophrenia, with loud, layered sounds and voices, and jarring camera work. When Lukas is at a point of experiencing an episode, the film switches from colour to black-and-white. As one reviewer observed:

Then as you start to recognize the 'symptoms' you virtually feel as if you yourself are experiencing the attack. It was very frightening. The middle-aged man sitting next to me during the screening, for example, hunched over his head between his knees every time an attack started.

In Frankfurt, the Düsseldorf Local Action Group used both films as part of an anti-stigma intervention and investigated data on the effectiveness of two very different styles of presentation. The group hosted two cinema shows and two panel discussions with individuals living with schizophrenia, medical professionals, and the director of *Das Weiße Rauschen*. Roughly one thousand people – ranging in age from 13 to 98 years of age, with a median age of 31 – attended. Fifty-seven per cent of those attending were female and 43% were male.

Roughly 149 of those in attendance responded to pre- and post-tests on knowledge and attitudes. In their self-assessment, 98% reported that they felt better informed about schizophrenia and 94% believed that they had a better understanding about people living with schizophrenia. Roughly nine of ten (91%) said they empathized more with the people with schizophrenia.

However, when asked questions about specific aspects of the illness and individuals diagnosed with schizophrenia, the results were more complex. Significantly more people reported that they would 'be able to maintain a friendship' with someone with schizophrenia (74.8%, pre-test; 89.1%, post-test). However, when asked about marrying someone with schizophrenia, 23% responded they would *not* consider marrying someone with schizophrenia in the pre-test; in the post-test 31.6% responded they would not.

Overall, when effects were compared between the two films, it was found that both films heightened the awareness and increased the knowledge of the illness. However, these films can also increase fear, negative attitudes and social distance. Having an opportunity to discuss the movies with people living with the illness helped further the understanding and reduce social distance.

When the two films were compared for their effectiveness in addressing stigma and discrimination, *A Beautiful Mind* – with its upbeat Hollywood conclusion – had a greater impact in reducing social distance.

Conclusion

Because many of the anti-stigma efforts described above are part of the German Research Network (supported by the Federal Ministry of Education and Research), national results of these efforts will be part of research presented in 2005/2006. However, preliminary research has already pointed to the importance of four elements.

The importance of focus groups in providing qualitative data (e.g. the specific content of stigmatizing language and behaviour, as well as the subjective experience of the stigmatized) that supplements quantitative data on knowledge and attitudes.

The potential for transnational/transcultural stigma work, such as the documentary films developed between the groups in Leipzig, Germany and Michalovce, Slovakia. This is being enhanced further by technological innovations such as the use of the Internet and low-cost digital video production. In addition a joint research project between Düsseldorf, Germany and Skopje, Macedonia is investigating difference between health care systems between the countries.

As with the interventions in Canada, the Local Action Groups in most German centres sought to balance carefully targeted interventions (such as those to high school students or mental health professionals) with broader, more 'public' activities such as cinema presentations.

Of the 20 WPA programmes underway internationally, several of the German Local Action Groups are notable for their close working relationship with consumer organizations such as BASTA and Irrsinnig Menschlich. These groups are actively involved in further empowering individuals living with schizophrenia socially and politically.

For more information on the Global Programme in Germany, please contact

- Anja Baumann (Coordinator)
  Department of Psychiatry, Heinrich-Heine-University Düsseldorf
  Bergische Landstr. 2
  40629 Düsseldorf, Germany
  Phone: (+49-211) 922 2777
  Fax: (+49-211) 922 2020
  E-mail: baumanna@uni-duesseldorf.de
- Wolfgang Gaebel (Advisor)
  Department of Psychiatry, Heinrich-Heine-University Düsseldorf
  Bergische Landstr. 2
  40629 Düsseldorf, Germany
  Phone: (+49-211) 922 2000
  Fax: (+49-211) 922 2020
  E-mail: wolfgang.gaebel@uni-duesseldorf.de

REFERENCES – GERMANY

Endicott, J., Spitzer, R.L., Fleiss, J.L. and Cohen, J. (1976). The Global Assessment Scale: a procedure of measuring overall severity of psychiatric disturbance. *Archives of General Psychiatry*, **33**, 766–771.

Kaiser, W. and Priebe, S. (1999). The impact of the interviewer–interviewee relationship on subjective quality of life ratings in schizophrenia patients. *International Journal of Social Psychiatry*, **45**(4), 292–301.

Link, B.G., Cullen, F.T., Struening, E., Shrout, P.E. and Dohrenwend, B.P. (1989). A modified labeling theory approach to mental disorders: an empirical assessment. *American Sociological Review*, **54**, 400–423.

Wahl, O.F. (1999). Mental health consumer's experience of stigma. *Schizophrenia Bulletin*, **25**, 467–478.

BIBLIOGRAPHY – GERMANY

Angermeyer, M.C. (2002). From intuition to evidence-based anti-stigma interventions. *World Psychiatry*, **16**(1), 1.

Angermeyer, M.C. and Matschinger, H. (2003). The stigma of mental illness: effects of labelling on public attitudes towards people with mental disorder. *Acta Psychiatrica Scandinavica*, **108**(4), 304–309.

Angermeyer, M.C. and Richter-Werling, M. (2003). [A mental health education program: the school project 'Crazy? So What!' initiated by 'Irrsinnig Menschlich (Madly Human) e.V. Leipzig'.] [German] 'Verruckt? Na und!' Ein Schulprojekt sensibilisiert Jugendliche fur psychische Probleme. *MMW Fortschritte der Medizin*, **145**(12), 38, 40–41.

Angermeyer, M.C., Schulze, B. and Dietrich, S. (2003). Courtesy stigma – a focus group study of relatives of schizophrenia patients. *Social Psychiatry and Psychiatric Epidemiology*, **38**(10), 593–602.

Angermeyer, M.C., Beck, M., Dietrich, S. and Holzinger, A. (2004a). The stigma of mental illness: patients' anticipations and experiences. *International Journal of Social Psychiatry*, **50**(2), 153–162.

Angermeyer, M.C., Buyantugs L., Kenzine, D.V. and Matschinger, H. (2004b). Effects of labelling on public attitudes towards people with schizophrenia: are there cultural differences? *Acta Psychiatrica Scandinavica*, **109**(6), 420–425.

Baumann, A., Zaeske, H. and Gaebel, W. (2003). [The image of people with mental illness in movies: effects on beliefs, attitudes and social distance, considering as example the movie 'The white noise'.] [German] Das Bild psychisch Kranker im Spielfilm: Auswirkungen auf Wissen, Einstellungen und soziale Distanz am Beispiel des Films 'Das weisse Rauschen'. *Psychiatrische Praxis*, **30**(7), 372–378.

Bock, T. and Naber, D. (2003). ['Anti-stigma campaign from below' at schools – experience of the initiative 'Irre menschlich Hamburg e.V.'.] [German]. Antistigmakampagne von unten – an Schulen – Erfahrungen der Initiative 'Irre menschlich Hamburg'. *Psychiatrische Praxis*, **30**(7), 402–408.

Davidson, M. (2002). What else can we do to combat stigma? *World Psychiatry*, **16**(1), 1.

Dietrich, S., Beck, M., Bujantugs, B., Kenzine, D., Matschinger, H. and Angermeyer, M.C. (2004). The relationship between public causal beliefs and social distance toward mentally ill people. *Australian and New Zealand Journal of Psychiatry*, **38**(5), 348–354; discussion 355–357.

Gaebel, W. (1999). [XI World Congress for Psychiatry. Hamburg, Germany, 6–11 August 1999.] [German] XI Weltkongress fur Psychiatrie. Hamburg, 6–11 August 1999. *Nervenarzt*, **70**(11), 1038–1039.

Gaebel, W. and Baumann, A.E. (2003a). Interventions to reduce the stigma associated with severe mental illness: experiences from the open the doors program in Germany. *Canadian Journal of Psychiatry – Revue Canadienne de Psychiatrie*, **48**(10), 657–662.

Gaebel, W. and Baumann, A.E. (2003b). ['Open the Doors' – the antistigma program of the World Psychiatric Association.] [German]. 'Open the Doors': Weltweite Initiative gegen die Stigmatisierung psychisch Kranker. *MMW Fortschritte der Medizin*, **145**(12), 34–37.

Gaebel, W., Baumann, A. and Witte, M. (2002a). [Attitude of the population to schizophrenic patients in 6 federal German large cities.] [German]. Einstellungen der Bevölkerung gegenüber schizophren Erkrankten in sechs bundesdeutschen Großstädten. *Nervenarzt*, **73**(7), 665–670.

Gaebel, W., Baumann, A., Witte, M. and Zäske, H. (2002b). Public attitudes towards people with mental illness in six German cities. Results of a public survey under special consideration of schizophrenia. *European Archives of Psychiatry and Clinical Neuroscience*, **252**(6), 278–287.

Schneider, F., Harter, M., Kratz, S., Bermejo, I., Mulert, C., Hegerl, U., Gaebel, W. and Berger, M. (2003). [Subjectively-perceived inappropriate treatment of depressed patients in general and psychiatric practice.] [German]. Unzureichender subjektiver Behandlungsverlauf bei depressiven Patienten in der haus- und nervenarztlichen Praxis. *Zeitschrift fur Arztliche Fortbildung und Qualitatssicherung*, **97**(Suppl. 4), 57–66.

Schulze, B. and Angermeyer, M.C. (2003). Subjective experiences of stigma. A focus group study of schizophrenic patients, their relatives and mental health professionals. *Social Science and Medicine*, **56**(2), 299–312.

Wahl, O.F. (1999). Telling is Risky Business: The Experience of Mental Illness Stigma. New Brunswick, Rutgers University Press.

Wolwer, W., Buchkremer, G., Hafner, H., Klosterkotter, J., Maier, W., Moller, H.J. and Gaebel, W. (2003). German research network on schizophrenia-bridging the gap between research and care. *European Archives of Psychiatry and Clinical Neuroscience*, **253**(6), 321–329.

6

Italy

Speaking at an international conference about the World Psychiatric Association (WPA) anti-stigma programme undertaken in Italy, Dr Giuseppe Rossi told the following story: Dr Richard Warner, Chairman of the Programme's Stigma Committee, had come to Brescia to consult with the Local Action Group. 'We presented Dr Warner with all the research we had done, all of the surveys we had conducted, studies of high school students, of journalists. We showed him all of the tabulated results, then asked him for his recommendations. He said: "I recommend you start doing something besides research."'

The local programme coordinator, Dr Giuseppe Rossi, is a psychiatrist in a hospital of the 'Centro San Giovanni di Dio' Fatebenefratelli. The Order of Saint John of God is a network of 250 Catholic hospitals in 48 countries. The order was founded in Grenada, Spain in the sixteenth century by John Cuidad. According to legend, he was a bookseller who had become a patient in the psychiatric wing of the city's Royal Hospital. After his release from the hospital, a friend let him stay on a small porch to escape the bitter cold winter. John Cuidad began taking in the poor and infirm who had no shelter.

Those involved in the programme at the hospital, planned, if the anti-stigma effort was successful, to extend the programme throughout the international organization and have it serve as a model for other hospitals in communities around the world. When Professors Sartorius and Lopez-Ibor met with the Head of the Order in Rome, he expressed considerable interest in the idea of expanding throughout the community of hospitals.

The Local Action Group assembled by Dr Rossi included: two psychiatrists, a psychologist, an official from the local health care system, a schoolteacher, a journalist, a local business owner, as well as a consumer and family member from Associazione Italiana Tutela Saluta Mentale, a national association of family members.

As with programs described earlier, the initiative in Brescia was announced to the media at a major press event. Eli Lilly and Company provided funding for the event and support for the 'Reintegration Awards', a programme launched to recognize excellence in rehabilitation work, in collaboration with the Italian Association of Psychiatry.

Research

The Brescia Local Action Group first surveyed 280 members of the general public using several different instruments:

- Community Attitudes to the Mentally Ill (CAMI) Inventory (Taylor and Dear, 1981).
- Fear And Behavioural Intentions (FABI) Inventory (Wolff *et al.*, 1996a).
- Semi-structured Interview (Wolff *et al.*, 1996b).

The group also conducted pre- and post-tests of the knowledge and attitudes of high school students before and after presentations given by a psychiatrist and psychologist. By the end of 2002, about 500 students had been surveyed.

A series of six focus group discussions were also organized – three with individuals living with schizophrenia, three with family members – to better understand the experience of stigma of mental illness by those directly affected by it. Forty individuals participated in the research (described below). Working with Beate Schulze from the Leipzig Local Action Group, the Brescia team compiled the data using a computer program called WinMax.

On the basis of this data, the Local Action Group developed interventions and messages for key target groups. In 1999, the group identified high school students, people living with schizophrenia and family members for their initial work. Once these efforts were successfully underway, in 2001, the programme selected two public target groups – employers and journalists – for anti-stigma activities.

Stigma and high school students

One of the first anti-stigma interventions undertaken by the Brescia group involved high school students. An experimental group of students from 16 to 18 years of age was identified in the urban area of Brescia. A control group of 186 subjects was also identified. These groups were selected at random from the last three school years of six schools (one teachers' training school, two lyceums, one technical school, one school specializing in scientific studies and one specializing in classical studies).

The Local Action Group secured permission from the provincial education office to conduct the research, before approaching the headmasters of the selected secondary schools. The students' knowledge and attitudes were measured using a questionnaire based on the Canadian survey. Students were given these questionnaires prior to the intervention and again 1 and 3 months after the 2½-h educational programme.

Before starting work with the students, the psychiatrist and psychologist team met with the teachers. In this initial 1-h presentation, teachers received information on mental illness, the stigma associated with mental illness and the goal of both the local education programme and the objectives of the WPA global anti-stigma programme. Each teacher was given two brochures:

- The first was a general overview of the myths and misunderstandings regarding mental illness and information designed to address negative stereotypes.
- The second was a more detailed and specific presentation of mental illnesses, their causes and their treatment.

The presentations to students were 2½ h in length. In these presentations, a consumer joined the psychiatrist and psychologist. Together the team presented information on a wide range of topics including aetiology and treatment of psychiatric disorders, as well as issues of stigma and discrimination. Students watched a videotape on the WPA global anti-stigma programme and were given a brochure on the local initiative in Brescia.

The control group of students did not participate in the intervention and did not receive any information about mental illness or the stigma associated with it. Both groups were then asked to complete survey instruments measuring knowledge and attitudes.

The results showed significant changes in attitudes towards people suffering from mental illness. Students in the experimental group were more willing to accept someone with mental illness in their class after the intervention. This same group of students also expressed less fear in speaking with someone suffering from a mental illness. The intervention team speculates that this reduction in fear is directly based on already having had a personal interaction with an individual with mental illness.

Stigma and journalists

This particular target group has proven to be challenging for the Brescia team. While the Calgary intervention had been able to achieve greater reach into the community of journalists by including a member in their group, the journalist on the Brescia Local Action Group was not able to establish a broader network of colleagues. In 2003, the group approached other journalists to have them assist in the intervention.

In 1998, focus groups with journalists were conducted to assess knowledge and attitudes. The Local Action Group also sought a deeper understanding of the origins of stereotypes and ways in which negative images are perpetuated in the media. Based on the results of these focus groups, the Local Action Group created a media kit and series of articles to better educate journalists about schizophrenia, and the stigma and discrimination associated with it.

The group conducted a pre-intervention survey of one of the leading newspapers *Il Giornale di Brescia* in 1998. Articles were evaluated as to the negative and positive images portrayed regarding mental illness.

In 2002, a second evaluation, using the same criteria, was undertaken. In the 4 years during which the anti-stigma effort was undertaken, the number of articles presenting positive messages of recovery and available treatment had increased. While the group believes its efforts have had some impact on this change, it continues its analysis into the many different reasons the shift may have occurred in the media.

Working with employers and their employees

The Local Action Group contacted 39 companies in the manufacturing sector of the province of Brescia. Government legislation requires that companies hire individuals with handicaps. The group administered questionnaires to the employers of each of these firms as well as 15 of their employees. In total 284 questionnaires were completed by employees and 39 by employers. Given the size of the employer sample it is difficult to show results with statistical significance.

However, the clearest trend, which was demonstrated with statistical significance, was that those business owners who had been in business and hiring employees the longest showed the most negative attitudes to the idea of employing individuals with mental illness.

Among the employees, a direct correlation was shown between the age of the employee and attitudes towards those with mental illness. Older workers had less positive attitudes toward people with schizophrenia than the young. Attitudes toward those with mental illness were more positive in companies where employees worked with individuals with disabilities. Similarly, the research showed that those who knew a colleague with mental illness were more likely to have positive attitudes.

After the first study exploring the attitudes of employers and employees toward people suffering from psychiatric disabilities, the Local Action Group analysed the previous 5 years of activities of NIL, a public agency providing supported employment services for those with disabilities. One unit within that agency is dedicated to employment issues for those with mental illness.

From 1998 to 2003, the unit tracked the employment of 70 people with serious mental illness. The percentage of those who have been employed and maintain their work is more than 30%. With that data, the Local Action Group has begun to assess levels of satisfaction among those who have received support – and their overall assessment of social integration. This study will be followed by an analysis of the family members and relatives. The final phase will then be an analysis of the employers themselves regarding the services provided by NIL.

The Brescia group will continue to use this data in its efforts to integrate those with mental illness into the workforce.

Focus group findings in Brescia

Following her work on focus groups with the intervention in Leipzig, Germany, the Brescia team asked Beate Schulze to assist them in a similar effort. Many of the same techniques and measurement instruments were used.

Six focus groups were organized: three with individuals living with schizophrenia and three with family members. Groups varied in size from six to eight participants. A total of 26 individuals diagnosed with schizophrenia (ICD-10) and 22 family members participated (eight mothers, four fathers, six sisters, three brothers and one husband). Of the individuals living with the illness, 75% were inpatients of the psychiatric rehabilitation residential care unit. The remaining 25% were outpatients of the same unit.

Overall, the experience of stigma and discrimination described by both groups differed in significant areas.

Experiences of stigma during the course of psychiatric treatment accounted for 36.5% of all experiences reported by family members. These relatives cited inadequacy of services and shortages of effective treatment, as well as an overall lack of respect and collaboration from the health care professionals.

Those living with schizophrenia, by contrast, complained about mental health services in only 7.5% of the examples of stigma and discrimination cited. They reported negative attitudes and prejudice of the community in 28.8% of the examples. Family members cited these examples in only 1.3% of the incidents.

One-fourth (24.8%) of the family members reported that stigma contributed to their own negative self-image, while describing the impact of social stigma on their own self-image in only 7.5% of the cases. However, nearly one-fifth of those living with schizophrenia expressed a concern about the lack of understanding of the illness by the general public (compared to 1.3% of relatives' accounts).

In the area of health care services, another interesting disparity occurred. Both individuals living with schizophrenia and their family members complained about the lack of services available and the distance they were required to travel to reach these services on the outskirts of town. However, relatives reported that they were not consulted on the treatment regimen of the family members and that doctors did not listen to them. They felt doctors did not appreciate their input into the care of the patient living in their household.

For example, they report that the doctor's recommendations are often at odds with what they feel they can do or provide. They were given little guidance in how to care for the individual and were told they simply 'must tolerate' the burden of the illness.

Overall, the qualitative research found that those living with schizophrenia and their family members consider stigma a major obstacle to reintegration into the community. At the same time, they acknowledge that they themselves may contribute to the process of stigmatization by accepting the public stereotypes and anticipating rejection based on those stereotypes.

The study also highlighted the importance of health care professionals involving both their patients and their family members in a dialogue of care to ensure greater involvement and compliance. Both groups reported markedly negative stigma and prejudice from medical professionals.

The results of these focus groups have been shared in two courses presented for the Italian Association of Psychiatry and Psycho-social Rehabilitation. Overall, this investigation demonstrated that focus groups are effective in gathering important qualitative data on the experiences of those living with mental illness to the medical professionals who are treating them. Relieved of the defensive posturing that can occur in the doctor–patient or doctor–family dyad, professionals may better understand the challenges patients and their families face, and conversely, individuals living with schizophrenia and family members may feel more empowered to become active participants in the treatment.

Conclusion

The Local Action Group in Brescia continues its anti-stigma work. In addition, it has expanded its educational efforts to other parts of Italy, assisting and consulting with groups interested in implementing interventions of their own.

Unfortunately, the further expansion of the programme into other hospitals in the international network of the Order of Saint John of God has not happened. This is due in part to a reorientation of the hospital's mission and greater investment in laboratory and diagnostic apparatus, which has led to a reduction in the budget set aside by the hospital for anti-stigma work.

In 2003, the group began working with the Catholic Church in Italy. Twenty seminarians agreed to participate in a study of knowledge and attitudes among the clergy. The intent, in a country where the population is nearly 99% Catholic, is to add the clergy to the growing list of target audiences that include: high school students, individuals living with schizophrenia and family members, journalists and business owners.

For more information on the Global Programme in Italy, please contact

- Chiara Buizza
  IRCCS 'Centro San Giovanni Di Dio – Fatebenefrateli'
  Via Pilastroni 4, 25125 Brescia, Italy
  Phone: (+39-030) 3501 506
  Fax: (+39-030) 3533 513
  E-mail: wpa.irccs@oh-fbf.it
- Marco Ponteri
  IRCCS 'Centro San Giovanni Di Dio – Fatebenefrateli'
  Via Pilastroni 4, 25125 Brescia, Italy
  Phone: (+39-030) 3501 506
  Fax: (+39-030) 3533 513
  E-mail: mponteri@oh-fbf.it
- Giuseppe Rossi (Coordinator)
  IRCCS 'Centro San Giovanni Di Dio – Fatebenefrateli'
  c/o Ist. S. Cuore di Gesù
  Via Pilastroni 4, 25123 Brescia, Italy
  Phone: (+39-030) 3501 571
  Fax: (+39-030) 3533 513
  E-mail: irccs.fatebenefrateli@oh-fbf.it

REFERENCES – ITALY

aylor, S.M. and Dear, M. (1981). Scaling community attitudes toward the mentally ill. *Schizophrenia Bulletin*, **7**(2), 225–240.

olff, G., Pathare, S., Craig, T. and Leff, J. (1996a). Community attitudes to mental illness. *British Journal of Psychiatry*, **168**(2), 183–190.

olff, G., Pathare, S., Craig, T. and Leff, J. (1996b). Community knowledge of mental illness and reaction to mentally ill people. *British Journal of Psychiatry*, **168**(2), 191–198.

BIBLIOGRAPHY – ITALY

Casacchia, M., Rossi, G. and Pioli, R. (2001). Schizofrenia e cittadinanza. Il Pensiero Scientifico Editore.

Magli, E., Buizza, C. and Pioli, R. (2004). Malattia mentale e mass media: una indagine su un quotidiano locale. *Recenti Progressi in Medicina*, **94**(6).

Magliano, L., Fadden, G., Economou, M., Xavier, M., Held, T., Guarneri, M., Marasco, C., Tosini, P. and Maj, M. (1998). Social and clinical factors influencing the choice of coping strategies in relatives of patients with schizophrenia: results of the BIOMED I study. *Social Psychiatry and Psychiatric Epidemiology*, **33**(9), 413–419.

Magliano, L., Guarneri, M., Fiorillo, A., Marasco, C., Malangone, C. and Maj, M. (2001a). A multicenter Italian study of patients' relatives' beliefs about schizophrenia. *Psychiatric Services*, **52**(11), 1528–1530.

Magliano, L., Malangone, C., Guarneri, M., Marasco, C., Fiorillo, A. and Maj, M. (2001b). [The condition of families of patients with schizophrenia in Italy: burden, social network and professional support.] [Italian] La situazione delle famiglie dei pazienti con schizofrenia in Italia: carico familiare, risposte dei SSM, sostegno sociale. *Epidemiologia e Psichiatria Sociale*, **10**(2), 96–106.

Magliano, L., De Rosa, C., Guarneri, M., Cozzolino, P., Malangone, C., Marasco, C., Fiorillo, A. and Maj, M. (2002a). [Causes and psychosocial consequences of schizophrenia: opinions of mental health personnel.] [Italian]. Cause e conseguenze psicosociali della schizofrenia: le opinioni degli operatori dei SSM. *Epidemiologia e Psichiatria Sociale*, **11**(1), 35–44.

Magliano, L., Marasco, C., Fiorillo, A., Malangone, C., Guarneri, M. and Maj, M. (2002b). Working Group of the Italian National Study on Families of Persons with Schizophrenia. The impact of professional and social network support on the burden of families of patients with schizophrenia in Italy. *Acta Psychiatrica Scandinavica*, **106**(4), 291–298.

Magliano, L., De Rosa, C., Fiorillo, A., Malangone, C., Guarneri, M., Marasco, C. and Maj, M. (2003). [Psychosocial causes and consequences of schizophrenia: opinions of Italians.] [Italian.] Cause e conseguenze psicosociali della schizofrenia: le opinioni degli Italiani. *Epidemiologia e Psichiatria Sociale*, **12**(3), 187–197.

Magliano, L., De Rosa, C., Fiorillo, A., Malangone, C. and Maj, M. (2004a). National Mental Health Project Working Group. Perception of patients' unpredictability and beliefs on the causes and consequences of schizophrenia – a community survey. *Social Psychiatry and Psychiatric Epidemiology*, **39**(5), 410–416.

Magliano, L., Fiorillo, A., De Rosa, C., Malangone, C. and Maj, M. (2004b). Beliefs about schizophrenia in Italy: a comparative nationwide survey of the general public, mental health professionals, and patients' relatives. *Canadian Journal of Psychiatry – Revue Canadienne de Psychiatrie*, **49**(5), 322–330.

Mangili, E., Ponteri, M., Buizza, C. and Rossi, G. (2004). Atteggiamenti nei confronti delle disabilità e della malattia mentale nei luoghi di lavoro: una rassegna. *Epidemiologia e Psichiatria Sociale*, **13**(1), 29–46.

Rossi, A., Amaddeo, F., Bisoffi, G., Ruggeri, M., Thornicroft, G. and Tansella, M. (2002). Dropping out of care: inappropriate terminations of contact with community-based psychiatric services. *British Journal of Psychiatry*, **181**, 331–338.

Vezzoli, R., Archiati, L., Buizza, C., Pasqualetti, P., Rossi, G. and Pioli, R. (2001). Attitude towards psychiatric patients: a pilot study in a northern Italian town. *European Psychiatry: The Journal of the Association of European Psychiatrists*, **16**(8), 451–458.

Warner, R., de Girolamo, G., Belelli, G., Bologna, C., Fioritti, A. and Rosini, G. (1998). The quality of life of people with schizophrenia in Boulder, Colorado, and Bologna, Italy. *Schizophrenia Bulletin*, **24**(4), 559–568.

7

Greece

On 7 September 1999, an earthquake measuring 5.9 on the Richter scale struck the Greek capital of Athens. More than 143 people were killed and hundreds more injured. More than 40 buildings in the metropolitan area collapsed. The State Psychiatric Hospital was severely damaged and residents of the hospital had to be moved to other temporary housing. A number of patients were placed in nearby hotels.

While the relocation was not done in secrecy, when some local residents heard news reporting about a violent incident at one of the hotels, neighbours began to speak out in opposition to housing patients in the hotels. They brought the case to court in order to evict patients from the neighbourhood. The judge ruled against the protesting residents and in favour of those temporarily housed in the hotels.

Initial anti-stigma work was already underway in Greece, but the public controversy provided an opportunity to study issues involving stigma and discrimination. A face-to-face survey was conducted with 200 residents, employers and employees in three areas of Athens:

- Metaxourgio, where patients were relocated;
- Koliatsou where, 8 years earlier, mental health services had successfully been integrated into the community;
- Liossio, an area that shared the same socio-demographic profile of the two other centres, but lacked psychiatric services or a group home in the community.

The study showed that individuals who had more contact with the mentally ill had more positive attitudes towards them as well. A second survey was conducted on a national level of 1119 respondents over the age of 15. This face-to-face survey explored the attitudes, knowledge and beliefs of the general public.

The majority of those surveyed (81.3%) said that those diagnosed with schizophrenia have a split personality. Nearly three out of four respondents (74.6%) said that those living with schizophrenia were dangerous. Overall, the general public showed a low level of knowledge and a high level of social distance. High social distance was reported among those of lower socio-economic status, living in rural areas, with little education, little knowledge of schizophrenia and no reported personal contact with individuals with schizophrenia. While 51.2% of respondents were in favour of small group homes in the community, 19.9% were opposed – and slightly more than half (56.6%) said they would actively resist them being established.

The majority of all respondents said that television was their main source of information about schizophrenia. Media portrayals of those with schizophrenia were reported to be generally negative.

Compared to similar surveys on social distance done in Germany and Canada, social distance in Greece was considerably high.

Based on the results of these surveys, the Local Action Group decided on a two-pronged approach:

(a) to address issues of stigma broadly, through the media;
(b) to develop more focused interventions with specially tailored programmes that would promote personal contact with individuals living with schizophrenia.

The Local Action Group selected a number of target audiences, similar to those chosen in other countries: high school students and teachers, individuals living with schizophrenia and family members, and mental health professionals.

A unique national opportunity

A second event would significantly affect the reach and effectiveness of the programme. In 2002, Professor Costas Stefanis, a member of the global programme Steering Committee, was named Minister of Health in Greece.

In addition to his participation in the anti-stigma effort, the Greek Local Action Group included individuals from the Division of Mental Health, the Institute for Paedagogics, the Family Association for Mental Health, Consumer Associations, journalists and the media, as well as lobbyists and business professionals. These individuals formed a number of different committees:

- The *honorary committee* includes an archbishop, politicians, journalists, academicians, artists and individuals 'with key roles in the community to facilitate networking for the overall programme'.
- The *research committee* includes professionals who would make recommendations on research needs and would be responsible for implementing the survey on knowledge, beliefs and attitudes.
- The *communication committee* includes individuals charged with building an effective communication plan, targeting social groups, and developing innovative social marketing and public relations techniques.
- The *education committee* oversees the preparation of informational materials.

- The *intervention committee* supervises and coordinates direct contacts with state and municipal authorities.
- The *review committee* is charged with monitoring and evaluating the overall efforts of the group, and reporting to the core Local Action Group.

The Local Action Group selected a number of target audiences similar to those chosen by other initiatives already described: mental health professionals, individuals living with schizophrenia and family members, as well as high school students and teachers. Given the national scope of the programme, the group also sought to communicate its message broadly to the general public.

Once the first three volumes of World Psychiatric Association (WPA) Programme materials were translated, the initial planning was completed and interventions were undertaken with each of these groups.

Mental health professionals

From its earliest work in 1999, the Local Action Group has maintained a training initiative for those in the mental health profession. The first of these involved 180 nurses, social workers, occupational therapists and others working in residential settings.

This programme placed an emphasis on facts concerning schizophrenia, its aetiology and treatment. Based on pre- and post-test assessments of knowledge and attitudes, this approach has proven successful in dispelling misunderstandings that surround the illness.

Making stigma a European priority

During its presidency of the European Union, the presiding country can select a topic that it considers particularly important and present it for the consideration to the ministers of the European Union countries. Through the auspices of Professor Costas Stefanis, Greece selected the problem of stigma as the topic for a Ministerial Conference held in Athens in March 2003.

The result was the inclusion of the work against stigma among the topics the European Union and its ministers should address. The Ministerial Conference on mental health, in Helsinki in January 2005 included stigma as one of the priorities for health programmes across Europe.

Working with the media

Given the influence of journalists in presenting stories of mental illness to the general public, the Local Action Group has placed strong emphasis on correcting commonly held misconceptions and educating opinion leaders. A press conference was held at the start of the programme to present results of the surveys of knowledge and attitudes.

Since June 2001, the Local Action Group has collected press clippings of stories in the print media that refer to mental illness. These stories are coded and filed so that attitudes and stereotypes might be tracked. In one 20-week analysis, two mental health experts have categorized articles in five areas: general references, mental health services, schizophrenia, mood and anxiety disorders. They found that of the 204 articles collected in that time period, 10.3% of articles, and 22.2% of those concerning schizophrenia, were stigmatizing.

Negative stereotypes and stigmatizing language appear in a wide range of popular media – from news programmes to television sit-coms. The Local Action Group in Greece established a 'Stigma Watch' Programme. One hundred volunteers were then trained to monitor a variety of media sources, for example, of stigmatizing imagery and language regarding mental illness.

Volunteers contact journalists, editors, publishers, producers and broadcasters explaining how a particular article or programme was stigmatizing and reinforced negative stereotypes and prejudice. Key to this effort is providing the journalists and editors with accurate information and advising on how the damage might be corrected. To date most of the communication has been through letter writing.

One example is the response to the publishing of a book with the original French title of 'Le Dingue au Bistouri' or 'The Lunatic with a Lancet'. The Greek translation made the stigma a little more specific with 'The Schizo with the Lancet'. The group contacted the publisher and is seeking to have the book given a less stigmatizing title in its second edition.

Expanding the volunteer network

Volunteerism in Greece is, according to members of the Local Action Group, 'not particularly widespread, especially when it comes to the mental health field'. However, in addition to building the volunteer Stigma Watch Group, media coverage of the programme has generated an increase in the number of volunteers. Most of these volunteers have been unemployed psychologists who work with the Associations of Patients and Families and also staff the phone line service.

The phone line service has been extremely important given the distribution nationwide of so many pamphlets and information flyers. Established in September 2002, the service is available for those seeking information on schizophrenia, on the anti-stigma programme or any other mental-health-related issues.

Records were kept of the requests for information so that the group might better assess the most urgent needs. Requests identified needs chiefly in three areas:

1 About mental illness in general, the service available and issues surrounding welfare, finances, legislation and consumers' rights.
2 Improvement in existing services.
3 Empowerment and support for individuals living with schizophrenia and family members.

Stigma and the arts

Initial research with the Canadian Pilot Programme raised questions about the effectiveness of broad interventions to the 'general public'. Yet the experiences with other programmes such as the effort in Greece may indicate a need to reassess how we measure the impact of an anti-stigma campaign.

In Calgary, the post-test measure of attitudes undertaken 10 weeks after a radio campaign showed results that were inconclusive at best. However, in Greece, the initiative to the general public was clearly effective in helping to create a network of volunteers to assist in the anti-stigma efforts.

Similarly, a series of public events, involving the arts earned the programme a good deal of press, addressed the myths and misunderstandings surrounding mental illness in general and schizophrenia in particular. Like the programmes in Spain and Germany, the Greek Local Action Group organized a special event to coincide with the release of the film *A Beautiful Mind* in July 2002. Prominent political, social and intellectual figures attended a special screening of the film at a large cinema in Athens. The event was covered by the press. Stories from that coverage appeared on television, the radio and in the print media for the next several weeks.

The following March, another event was organized around the first staging in Greece of the play *Proof*. The play, which won a Pulitzer Prize in the US, has played internationally in New York, London and Paris. The drama concerns a young woman whose father, a professor of mathematics, suffered from an unspecified mental illness. During the course of the play, she seeks 'proof' of her own mathematical genius, the possibility of her own mental illness and her affections for a young grad student.

Actors, journalists and politicians were invited to a special performance of the play. A lively conversation, involving members of the audience, followed the performance. Actors, people living with schizophrenia and other attendees spoke in dramatic and sometimes emotional terms about schizophrenia and the stigma associated with it.

Later in 2003, two other major events were held. The first, a benefit concert, is described below. The second was a 4-day film festival on mental illness and stigma, part of the popular Thessaloniki Film Festival in November. Two halls were used for film screenings and a series of related cultural events. One criterion for the selection of the films was that each should deal in some way with the stigma and discrimination experienced by those with mental illness. Another was that it must address one of the commonly held myths regarding mental illness. The films were presented with discussions that included psychiatrists, film critics, directors, actors, as well as consumers of mental health services and family members.

The films selected fell into three categories:

1 Those dealing with stereotypes of violence (*Repulsion*; *Fight Club* and *Through a Glass, Darkly*).
2 The stigma experience in the family (*Shine*; *I am Sam* and *Frances*).
3 Issues of rehabilitation and social integration (*Girl, Interrupted*; *Elling* and *Angel Baby*).

The festival was intended as more than public education on mental illnesses, but as an investigation into the realities of mental illness, its treatment, the challenges of recovery, and the stigma and discrimination experienced by individuals.

Support materials for communication

The release of the film *A Beautiful Mind* provided an opportunity to further facilitate public dialogue on schizophrenia and the stigma associated with it. The Local Action Group prepared a six-page informational pamphlet using images from the movie. The pamphlet provided an overview of key facts about the illness, its associated stigma and the varieties of social discrimination.

More than 1,500,000 pamphlets were distributed in cooperation with the 10 largest newspapers in the country. Another 600,000 were distributed by volunteers at cinemas, theatres and videoclubs in Athens. An additional 1,700,000 were mailed out in the region of Attica, accompanying mailings from the national Water Company. Mental health services throughout Greece received more than 50,000 for distribution to individuals living with schizophrenia, families and friends. Another 30,000 have been distributed at conferences, workshops, academic institutions and non-governmental organizations (NGO).

In a country with a population of 10,000,000, more than 3.3 million pamphlets have been distributed. They have also been translated into Turkish, Albanian, Arabic and Kurdish to reach immigrant communities living and working in Greece.

Celebrity and stigma

If there is a cultural antithesis to the concept of stigma, it is celebrity. While stigma and discrimination can keep individuals from having a voice in society through homelessness, unemployment and other disenfranchisements, celebrity enables an individual to be heard by a wider audience, and perhaps provide a voice for those who are not allowed to speak, or who speak and are not heard.

In September 2003, the Local Action Group organized a concert at the Herodium Theatre in the shadows of the great Acropolis of Athens. Nana Mouskouri, an internationally renowned vocalist and supporter of the anti-stigma movement, was the featured performer. To show the international nature of the WPA anti-stigma movement, the evening's performance also featured John McDermott, a Canadian tenor with roots in Ireland and Scotland.

The high-profile event attracted well-known figures from politics, the cultural community and the psychiatric profession. Four awards were presented that evening: one to Nana Mouskouri, to the President of the Families Association for Mental Health, to the President of the Association of Patients, and the main sponsor of the international WPA Programme, Eli Lilly and Company.

Along with the usual information on the performers, sponsors and evening's selections of music, the playbill contained information about mental illness and the stigma associated with it, as well as an overview of the Stigma Watch Programme. Press coverage of the event was featured on television, the radio and in newspapers and magazines.

Moving forward, the WPA is working to enlist the support of other international celebrities to help spread the message of inclusion.

Stigma and high school students

In 2003, a nationwide educational initiative was undertaken in collaboration with the Greek Ministry of Education. The aim of this effort is to instil tolerance of diversity and respect for human rights for those living with mental illness. Stigma and the discrimination associated with it will be one of the core components of the curriculum.

Individuals living with schizophrenia and families

The Local Action Group established six psychoeducational programmes for relatives and four programmes for individuals living with schizophrenia. The training package included: videotapes, brochures and informational booklets about schizophrenia. As these programmes have been established, they can be easily replicated and extended further out into the community.

The work was done in collaboration with Associations of Patients and Families and included the creation of a seminar on the stigma associated with schizophrenia. A special family support group for those with relatives living with schizophrenia was also established.

Local networking and awareness

At the start of this chapter, we described the research undertaken following the Athens earthquake. Research indicated that those who had had contact with individuals with mental illness were likely to be more tolerant and have a greater positive attitude. In light of those findings, the Greek Local Action Group set up a programme designed to improve attitudes towards those living with mental illness.

The Local Action Group works in partnership with consumer and family organizations to organize presentations about schizophrenia in the community. The presentations are conducted with the support of the three main psychiatric hospitals of Athens and take place in neighbourhoods where group homes for those with mental illness already exist or are scheduled to be opened in the future. The goal is to establish a social support network within the community and creates a neighbourhood branch of the consumer–family associations.

Conclusion

To date, Greece is the only Local Action Group in the global programme to have one of its key participants elevated to Minister of Health of the country. Undoubtedly, the active involvement of such a major political figure did much to advance the anti-stigma effort in the country.

Having that opportunity, however, is not the same thing as effectively acting upon it and certainly every Local Action Group through the careful selection of its initial members has its own unique opportunities. As noted with other programmes, it is important to include members of your target audience in the Local Action Group. Other learning points from the Greek experience include:

- The building of a volunteer network to expand the reach of the programme, provide support for events in the community and assist in efforts such as the 'Stigma Watch'.
- The involvement of high-profile members of the community and celebrities to draw media attention to the effort.
- Recognizing that television was the primary medium through which people said they received information on schizophrenia, the Greek Local Action Group created public events to attract those community leaders and celebrities, and achieve a great deal of press coverage.

- Working in partnership with other groups is also important to the effective distribution of information and communication materials. Working with the Ministry of Education the group was able to establish a curriculum for high school students. Working with the utilities industry, the group effectively distributed hundreds of thousands of flyers to virtually every household in Greece.

The effort in Greece is an example of a programme that has been able to build national profile and maintain momentum. The programme continues on a national level as of this writing though there is a new Minister of Health.

For more information on the Global Programme in Greece, please contact

- Christina Aramandani
  University Mental Health Research Institute (UMHRI)
  Papagou, P.O. Box 66517
  156-01, Athens, Greece
  Phone: (0030-210) 6170822
  Fax: (0030-210) 6519796
  E-mail: stigma@compulink.gr
- Marina Economou (Coordinator)
  University Mental Health Research Institute (UMHRI)
  Papagou, P.O. Box 66517
  156-01, Athens, Greece
  Phone: (0030-210) 6170823
  Fax: (0030-210) 6519796
  E-mail: stigma@compulink.gr
- Costas Stefanis (Advisor)
  University Mental Health Research Institute (UMHRI), Eginition Hospital
  Athens University Medical School
  73–74, Vasilissis Sophias Avenue
  11528, Athens, Greece
  Phone: (0030-210) 7217763/6422025
  Fax: (0030-210) 7243905/7239805
  E-mail: iumhri@compulink.gr

BIBLIOGRAPHY – GREECE

Daskalopoulou, E.G., Dikeos, D.G., Papadimitriou, G.N., Souery, D., Blairy, S., Massat, I., Mendlewicz, J. and Stefanis, C.N. (2002). Self-esteem, social adjustment and suicidality in affective disorders. *European Psychiatry: The Journal of the Association of European Psychiatrists*, **17**(5), 265–271.

Madianos, M.G. and Economou, M. (1999). The impact of a Community Mental Health Center on psychiatric hospitalizations in two Athens areas. *Community Mental Health Journal*, **35**(4), 313–323.

Madianos, M.G., Madianou, D., Vlachonikolis, J. and Stefanis, C.N. (1987). Attitudes towards mental illness in the Athens area: implications for community mental health intervention. *Acta Psychiatrica Scandinavica*, **75**(2), 158–165.

Madianos, M.G., Economou, M. and Stefanis, C.N. (1998). Long-term outcome of psychiatric disorders in the community: a 13-year follow-up study in a nonclinical population. *Comprehensive Psychiatry*, **39**(2), 47–56.

Madianos, M.G., Economou, M., Hatjiandreou, M., Papageorgiou, A. and Rogakou, E. (1999). Changes in public attitudes towards mental illness in the Athens area (1979/1980–1994). *Acta Psychiatrica Scandinavica*, **99**(1), 73–78.

Magliano, L., Fadden, G., Economou, M., Xavier, M., Held, T., Guarneri, M., Marasco, C., Tosini, P. and Maj, M. (1998). Social and clinical factors influencing the choice of coping strategies in relatives of patients with schizophrenia: results of the BIOMED I study. Social *Psychiatry and Psychiatric Epidemiology*, **33**(9), 413–419.

Magliano, L., Fadden, G., Economou, M., Held, T., Xavier, M., Guarneri, M., Malangone, C., Marasco, C. and Maj, M. (2000). Family burden and coping strategies in schizophrenia: 1-year follow-up data from the BIOMED I study. *Social Psychiatry and Psychiatric Epidemiology*, **35**(3), 109–115.

Tomaras, V., Mavreas, V., Economou, M., Ioannovich, E., Karydi, V. and Stefanis, C. (2000). The effect of family intervention on chronic schizophrenics under individual psychosocial treatment: a 3-year study. *Social Psychiatry and Psychiatric Epidemiology*, **35**(11), 487–489.

8

United States

In 1999, the US Bureau of Justice Statistics estimated that 283,000 jail and prison inmates suffered from a serious mental illness. One in four female inmates is reported to have a mental illness. Nearly half of the mentally ill inmates had been imprisoned for a non-violent crime. Twenty per cent of those with mental illness (male and female) had been homeless during the year before their incarceration, according to a study by the Center for Mental Health Services. In 2003, Human Rights Watch reported: 'all-too-often seriously ill prisoners receive little or no meaningful treatment. They are neglected, accused of malingering, treated as disciplinary problems'.

Two other statistics further underscore the challenges for the mentally ill in the US. First, only 60% of the mentally ill in state and federal prisons reported receiving mental health treatment since incarceration. Second, the US remains one of the few countries in the world that executes the mentally ill if they commit a capital crime.

One explanation often given for such shocking statistics is that: in 1955, 560,000 men and women were in US State Psychiatric Hospitals; in 2004, there were fewer than 40,000. While the doors of institutions have been thrown open, public mental health services have been grossly inadequate to address the needs of the mentally ill.

The Local Action Group working in Boulder, Colorado sought to disrupt the vicious cycle that sweeps many of the mentally ill into the justice and penal systems where their illnesses continue to go untreated, and they emerge with a double stigma.

Boulder is 25 miles northwest of Denver, Colorado. Located in the Rocky Mountains, the city has a population of roughly 100,000 people, is home to the University of Colorado, and boasts 'more used bookstores per capita than any other City in the US'.

Professor Richard Warner, the head of the anti-stigma group in Boulder, has been chair of the Stigma Committee of the World Psychiatric Association (WPA) Global Programme. He also participated in the Pilot Programme in Canada and applied some of the lessons learned there to the efforts in Colorado.

While the results from the Canadian programme were being analyzed, Professor Warner organized a Local Action Group that included: psychiatrists, people living with schizophrenia and family members, a schoolteacher, a judge, a journalist and a representative from a local media agency. One of the first tasks was to conduct a survey to gain a better first-person perspective on stigma and discrimination.

Of the 56 individuals living with schizophrenia that were interviewed, 32 (66%) reported that stigma is a major, very severe or overwhelming problem in their lives. The groups seen as most stigmatizing are ranked here in descending order with the most stigmatizing first:

- employers or potential employers;
- general health physicians, emergency room staff and hospital staff;
- family members;
- police;
- television news and programmes, as well as newspaper reports;
- co-workers and neighbours;
- the general public.

A majority of family members also identified stigma as a major, very severe or overwhelming problem in their lives. The groups they identified were:

- family members;
- employers or potential employers;
- co-workers, friends and neighbours;
- newspapers and television;
- the general public.

Based upon these findings, the target groups selected were: employers; the media, including journalists; police and members of the criminal justice system. With experiences gained from working with the Partnership Programme in Calgary, the group also selected high school students as a way to change attitudes of the general public over time. In April 2000, Eli Lilly and Company awarded a financial grant to the campaign.

Employers

The Calgary group had encountered challenges in addressing this target group, in part, because they had not reached key change agents in the business community. For that reason, the Boulder Local Action Group met early in their planning process with the president of the Boulder Chamber of Commerce. Fifty per cent of all of the jobs in Boulder are with just 12 companies, including the University of Colorado. Developing a strategy to reach and mobilize these 12 companies was seen as having a great deal of potential for achieving change in employment.

Working with the Chamber of Commerce, the group developed an action plan for working with local employers. The Chamber President also supported a lunchtime educational presentation on discrimination against people with mental illness that was made to members.

In 1998, the University of Colorado, Boulder employed 6471 employees; a little less than one-third (1973) were instructors. Members of the Local Action Group met with the human resource department managers and employee assistance programme staff of the University. Working together with the anti-stigma group, the university employee assistance programme trained all university supervisors on the Boulder campus on issues related to mental illness in the workplace in March 2002. A month later, a workshop on mental illness was held at the diversity training programme for the university's administrative services.

In general terms, the approach taken with the Chamber of Commerce and efforts at the University of Colorado have yielded more substantive results than the Calgary and Brescia initiatives. The Local Action Group was able to meet with human resource directors and make presentations on mental illness and the effects of its stigma. Yet from the data available, employers remain one of the most stigmatizing groups and one of the most resistant to anti-stigma efforts.

Criminal justice system

Professionals in law enforcement and the judiciary often encounter people with mental illness in acute crisis situations. Surveys in Boulder showed that only a few of these professionals believed people with mental illness can recover from them.

Working together with the Local Action Group, the Chief Judge of the district court has held task force meetings with managers and leaders of all the local criminal justice agencies, including the judiciary, the county sheriff's department, the Boulder city police department, the county jail, the probation department, community corrections, the district attorney's office, the public defender's office, the mental health centre, the public health department and the alcohol recovery centre. The goal of the meetings has been to reduce the number of people with mental illness who are jailed. Police officers, other law enforcement personnel and members of the judiciary have received training on recognizing mental illness and have been given ways to deal more effectively with individuals in a crisis.

To date the anti-stigma efforts to this target audience have been extremely effective. Products of this group include:

• A new multi-agency community monitoring and treatment programme. The goal of the programme is to assist people living with schizophrenia with concomitant substance abuse problems and reduce the possibility they might end up in jail in the future.

• A training programme for professionals. Targeted to police officers, probation officers, corrections officers, attorneys and judges, the programme is designed to reduce fear of the mentally ill. After an initial pilot test with veteran and rookie police officers, the programme has been broadened to others.

Participants' knowledge scores improved substantially in pre/post-testing. The percentage of correct answers among veteran officers rose from 50% to 75%. Among new recruits, correct answers rose from 62% to 75%. However, initial pre/post-testing showed no improvements in attitudes toward the mentally ill.

A 4-h training course on adult and child mental health. This course was given to every member of the Longmont police force in April 2000. (Longmont is a city located in Boulder County, 16 miles from the City of Boulder.) The officers' scores on a pre/post-test on adult mental illness improved by 48%. The proportion of officers holding misconceptions about the causes of schizophrenia dropped from 24% to 3%, and the proportion holding misconceptions about the usual behaviour of people with schizophrenia dropped from 82% to 71%. The proportion with accurate information about when involuntary treatment could be initiated because of 'grave disability' improved from 48% to 71%.

With a faculty that included psychiatrists, individuals living with schizophrenia, and family members, individual classes were 90-min in length and were presented at the county justice centre to judges, magistrates, as well as public and private attorneys and probation officers. After the first training session on schizophrenia, knowledge scores improved by 58% and attitude scores improved by 17%. Judges requested further training on juvenile mental health issues and were provided with two additional 1-h sessions.

Members of the local action group also presented a criminal justice training programme at the annual meeting of the Colorado branch of the National Alliance for the Mentally Ill, to diffuse the training programme further into other communities. Criminal justice and mental health managers have also expressed interest in replicating the programme.

For that reason, an 8-h training curriculum on mental illness has been developed, targeted to police and corrections officers. The training course includes an instructor's guide and PowerPoint presentation and has been used in a number of communities in Colorado and other states.

Today, 90-min classes on mental illness continue to be taught at the county justice centre for judges, magistrates, probation officers, and public and private attorneys.

Media and the general public

Following lessons learned from the Calgary Pilot Programme, the Boulder Action Group also included a representative from one of the city's largest newspapers as one of its members. A media consultant was hired to work closely with the group.

A number of articles, editorials, letters and guest opinion columns have appeared in local newspapers on the anti-stigma campaign, the stigma of mental illness and other related issues. This included a front page article on stigma in the *Longmont Times-Call* newspaper.

The Local Action Group has provided journalists of all the Boulder County newspapers with a resource list of individuals living with schizophrenia, family members and professionals who can be called upon for information or background on a variety of mental health topics. This information packet also included suggestions for reducing stigma in reporting news and other stories that refer to mental illness.

During the initial implementation phase of the programme, as news spread through the community of the effort, call-in radio programmes have also dealt with the issues of stigma and prejudice. When Otto Wahl, the Director of the National Stigma Clearinghouse and author of *Media Madness* was invited to Boulder by the Local Action Group to give a public workshop on combating the stigma of mental illness in the media, he was also featured on one of these call-in programmes.

Working with the Department of Journalism of the University of Colorado, a content analysis of the *Boulder Daily Camera* is being conducted to assess media coverage before and after the campaign. Today, articles, editorials and letters continue to appear in the local media, keeping the public informed about the impact of stigma and discrimination on those living with mental illness.

High school students: reaching beyond schools

With assistance of on-site training from members of the Partnership Programme in Calgary, the Local Action Group in Boulder has developed a consumer speakers' bureau at the Mental Health Center of Boulder County. Consumer and family members are given training in public speaking and a representative from each group speaks to local high school classes.

In the fall semester of 1999, the speakers' bureau presented to 12 schools and community groups. In spring semester of 2000, the number rose to 17. In spring semester 2003, over 20 presentations were made. The speakers' bureau also presented to 400 students of Boulder High School at the World Affairs Conference Symposium.

In addition to improving the knowledge and attitudes of students, the group has been successful in having the Boulder Valley School District implement a new health curriculum for high school students.

Every year since 2000, an annual competition has been held in Boulder Valley high schools. Students are asked to produce anti-stigma materials in the form of posters and artwork. Winners have their artwork featured in displays throughout the community.

Indeed, it is the addition of communication materials *outside* the school that sets the Boulder Programme apart from the earlier effort in Calgary. Having narrowed the target audience from 'general public' to 'high school students', the Local Action Group delivered targeted messages in two media: on transit cards in city buses and as presentation slides in local cinemas during the summer months.

Cinemas. Cinemas become an even more popular destination for teenagers in the summertime when school is not in session. For that reason, for 3 months in the summer of 2002, slides with anti-stigma messages were featured before and after presentations in two local theatres – with a total of 16 screens.

Eighteen per cent of cinema patrons exiting the cinemas could recall one or more of the messages. Given the attendance at theatres during the 3 month period (roughly 60,000), approximately 11,000 people would have been able to recall a positive message. With the relatively modest costs of this medium (relative to radio or television advertising), the reach of the messages to the entire audience is pennies per viewer.

Transit cards/outdoor advertising. For the first 3 months of 2002, transit cards featuring anti-stigma messages were on display on 50 Boulder buses. The routes selected were those travelled by students on their way to high school or college. The theme of these transit cards were that: 'mental illness does not equal violence'.

Based upon interest in the messages and the relative low cost of the medium, additional transit cards were created. These cards featured winning entries from the high school art competition.

Research was not conducted on the cumulative effects of these messages on the community. However, given the wide distribution of these media, many teenagers whose knowledge and attitudes were improved through in-class speakers' bureau presentations, saw those anti-stigma messages reinforced in the community – at the movies they attended and on the buses they rode.

Conclusion

The development of training of law enforcement officials is an iterative process. Among some of the important lessons Richard Warner and the Local Action Group learned was the importance of particular topics such as suicide and why people with personality disorders are often not admitted to hospital. 'Because they may not recognize symptoms of mental illness and how these relate to suicide attempts, police officers,' Dr Warner explains, 'are likely to complain about a patient whom they brought in for evaluation after a suicide attempt – was treated, then released. They will tell us: "She got home before I did"'. Understanding the reasons behind a psychiatrist's decision to discharge a patient can also address some of the stigma these officers may feel toward the medical establishment.

They also learned the importance of the endorsement and presence of the police chief and other senior officers in sending a message about the value of the training. (Often these senior officials are not present during training of the night shift.)

Most important of all is the involvement of people living with the illness in the training. For many officers the only exposure they may have had with individuals with mental illness is in a crisis situation. This is true for members of the judiciary as well. Not only did knowledge of schizophrenia improve from 47% to 74% after the presentations, some judges reported immediate changes in their sentencing practices for adults and juveniles.

More information and training resources are available on-line at: www.mhcbc.org.

For more information on the Global Programme in United States, please contact

- Richard Warner (Coordinator)
  Mental Health Center of Boulder County
  1333 Iris Ave
  Boulder, Colorado 80302, USA
  Phone: (+1-303) 443 8500
  Fax: (+1-303) 449 6029
  E-mail: drdickwarner@aol.com

BIBLIOGRAPHY – UNITED STATES

Corrigan, P.W. (2004). Don't call me nuts: an international perspective on the stigma of mental illness. *Acta Psychiatrica Scandinavica*, **109**(6), 403–404.

Priebe, S., Warner, R., Hubschmid, T. and Eckle, I. (1998). Employment, attitudes toward work, and quality of life among people with schizophrenia in three countries. *Schizophrenia Bulletin*, **24**(3), 469–477.

Thompson, A.H., Stuart, H., Bland, R.C., Arboleda-Florez, J., Warner, R., Dickson, R.A., Sartorius, N., Lopez-Ibor, J.J., Stefanis, C.N., Wig, N.N. and WPA, World Psychiatric Association (2002). Attitudes about schizophrenia from the pilot site of the WPA worldwide campaign against the stigma of schizophrenia. *Social Psychiatry & Psychiatric Epidemiology*, **37**(10), 475–482.

Wahl, O.F. (1999). Mental health consumers' experience of stigma. *Schizophrenia Bulletin*, **25**(3), 467–478.

Wahl, O.F. and Harman, C.R. (1989). Family views of stigma. *Schizophrenia Bulletin*, **15**(1), 131–139.

Wahl, O.F. and Kaye, A.L. (1992). Mental illness topics in popular periodicals. *Community Mental Health Journal*, **28**(1), 21–28.

Wahl, O.F. and Lefkowits, J.Y. (1998). Impact of a television film on attitudes toward mental illness. *American Journal of Community Psychology*, **17**(4), 521–528.

Warner, R. (1999a). Environmental interventions in schizophrenia. 1: the individual and the domestic levels. *New Directions for Mental Health Services*, **83**, 61–70.

Warner, R. (1999b). Environmental interventions in schizophrenia. 2: the community level. *New Directions for Mental Health Services*, **83**, 71–84.

Warner, R. (1999c). Reducing the stigma associated with schizophrenia. In: Maj, M., ed. *Evidence and Experience in Psychiatry: Volume 2, Schizophrenia*. John Wiley & Sons, New York, pp. 284–286.

Warner, R. (1999d). Schizophrenia and the environment: speculative interventions. *Epidemiologia e Psichiatria Sociale*, **8**(1), 19–34.

Warner, R. (2000). *The Environment of Schizophrenia: Innovations in Practice, Policy and Communications*. London: Routledge (Lithuanian edition, 2003. Russian and Greek editions, 2004).

Warner, R. (2001a). Combating the stigma of schizophrenia. *Epidemiologia e Psichiatria Sociale*, **10**(1), 12–17.

Warner, R. (2001b). Community attitudes towards mental disorder. In: Thornicroft, G. and Szmukler, G., eds. *Textbook of Community Psychiatry*. Oxford University Press, Oxford.

Warner, R. (2001c). The prevention of schizophrenia: what interventions are safe and effective? *Schizophrenia Bulletin*, **27**(4), 551–562.

Warner, R. (2003). How much of the burden of schizophrenia is alleviated by treatment? *British Journal of Psychiatry*, **183**, 375–376.

Warner, R. (2004). Recovery form Schizophrenia: Psychiatry and Political Economy, 3rd edn. Brunner-Routledge, Hove and New York.

Warner, R. and Mandiberg, J.M. (2003). Changing the environment of schizophrenia at the community level. *Australasian Psychiatry*, **11**(Suppl.)

Warner, R., de Girolamo, G., Belelli, G., Bologna, C., Fioritti, A. and Rosini, G. (1998). The quality of life of people with schizophrenia in Boulder, Colorado, and Bologna, Italy. *Schizophrenia Bulletin*, **24**(4), 559–568.

9

Poland

On 15 September, 2002, an archway – festooned with flowers and garland – stood in the central square in Kraków, Poland. Those in the crowd who had come to celebrate the first Day of Solidarity with People Suffering from Schizophrenia were invited to step through the doorway and sign a petition affirming their solidarity to those living with schizophrenia.

Similar events were held in 15 other cities around Poland, including Warsaw. One hundred and eighty-seven media outlets – newspapers, magazines, radio and television – covered the nationwide celebration.

In 2003, the event had doubled in size. Thirty-two cities held public exhibitions: art displays, poetry readings and theatre performances by individuals living with schizophrenia.

That same month, the Polish Ministry of Health named the 'Open the Doors' programme the 'Success of the Year in Health Care'. The work begun by Dr Andrzej Cechnicki and Anna Bielañska in 2000 has evolved into one of the most successful national efforts in the global World Psychiatric Association (WPA) programme.

Putting the structure in place

Poland is a nation of roughly 38.5 million people, covering 312,685 km^2. A national anti-stigma effort that far-reaching requires careful coordination of many people. In March 2000, a core team of four professionals, including Dr Cechnicki and Ms Bielañska of Jagiellonian University in Kraków, held its first meeting with 15 individuals from eight different regions of the country. These team members included professionals and members of family organizations.

Regular monthly meetings were key to the coordination of the different regions. Similar in style to the monthly meetings held in the more localized Calgary initiative, the group would review progress and set new objectives for the future.

Another important element was the support of the Polish Ministry of Health, the Ministry of Work and Social Care, the Polish Psychiatric Association, and Eli Lilly and Company. Working in cooperation with these groups, the Polish team established a four-step plan for its nationwide effort. The success of each step was in part dependent on the successful implementation of the one that came before:

1 Assess the needs of individuals living with schizophrenia and family members to identify areas of stigma and discrimination.
2 Prepare information about schizophrenia and the stigma associated with it. This approach presents the perspectives of the consumer, family and mental health professionals to be distributed nationally to both print and broadcast journalists.
3 Develop an educational programme based on the experiences of individuals living with schizophrenia and professionals, including psychiatrists, teachers, journalists, priests and clerics.
4 Hold a series of symposia on schizophrenia at both the national and local levels, bringing together psychologists, general practitioners, social workers, people living with schizophrenia and family members.

Assessing needs

A number of surveys have been conducted in the first 4 years of the initiative in Poland, using both qualitative and quantitative methods.

The first round of research included focus group interviews with people living with schizophrenia and family members. While the information collected gave Local Action Group members first-hand accounts of the stigma experienced by those living with schizophrenia, the data was somewhat limited in scope and its applicability to the programme. In 2004, in the southern Malopolska region of Poland, the subjective experiences of a larger group of 200 individuals were investigated.

In 2001, Jacek Wciórka and Bogda Wciórka organized a national survey of public attitudes towards those with mental illness. The researchers sought to investigate:

• the public's understanding of the term 'schizophrenia';
• the degree to which is it used in the social experience;
• the social perception and position of schizophrenia;
• factors which might affect how individuals view medical treatment of the illness and the social climate that surrounds individuals diagnosed with the illness.

The research team, working with CBOS (Public Opinion Research Center), sampled 1000 adults from all over Poland. Individuals were selected at random and interviewed by telephone.

The survey found that the majority of the general public lacked sufficient information and knowledge about schizophrenia, and had negative stereotypes of those living with the illness. Most expressed stigmatizing beliefs (e.g. people with schizophrenia are violent) and held overall ambivalent feelings towards those with mental illness.

In July 2003, a study of the opinions of young Poles (ages 15–35 years) was conducted. A number of clear conclusions could be drawn about this group:

- Roughly one in four reported that they knew nothing about schizophrenia.
- The self-reported level of social acceptance of those with schizophrenia was high; a majority declared openness and support for those living with the illness.
- Those with higher education (18%) and living in larger metropolitan areas (22%) had better knowledge about the illness.
- Individuals with elementary school education (34%) and living in smaller villages (33%) reported no knowledge about the illness.
- A majority of young Poles knew little about the age groups typically at risk and were unaware that first symptoms appear in younger adults.
- 80% reported that those living with schizophrenia should not be isolated and that if properly treated, they can return to the community.

Overall social distance was small with a majority being open to individuals with schizophrenia living in their neighbourhood, and said that they would study, work and socialize with those having a mental illness.

While reporting that they would like to know more about the illness, 49% said they wanted the information to come from television compared to 41% reporting they wanted their information from newspapers, and 24% interested in learning about the illness from a meeting with someone with the illness. Only 17% reported wanting to learn about it in school or university.

A national perspective

The national programme in Poland approached the challenge of covering the country using a strategy different from that used in other programmes. The National Steering Committee of four and the fifteen regional representatives developed a series of programmes and agreed to replicate each in different cities or regions after initial pilot testing in one or two towns or villages. The result is a programme that has gradually built up a consistent momentum over time.

A non-governmental organization dedicated to schizophrenia

'Open the Door' is the name of the non-governmental organization (NGO) of individuals living with schizophrenia that was established in Poland. The goal of this NGO was education of those living with schizophrenia and their families. The group also seeks to educate professionals and other social groups.

Presentations to these groups focus on issues affecting the lives of people living with schizophrenia. These presentations allow individuals living with the illness to share information with other consumers on the illness itself and on the self-stigma that can keep many from taking a more active role in their treatment. Professionals often participate in these seminars and some of these presentations involve lessons the medical professional has learned from hearing the stories of people who live with the illness about the stigma and discrimination they experience first hand.

The overall goals of the 'Open the Door' Association are:

- to increase the number of educational seminars at psychiatric conferences regarding the subjective experience of illness and recovery;
- to become educators for politicians, clergy and other groups at seminars about mental health problems on the local and national levels;
- to increase participation of NGO spokespersons in the press, as well as in radio and television.

A national magazine produced by individuals living with schizophrenia entitled '*For Us*' further helps unify the national effort. The magazine contains stories of those living with schizophrenia, as well as resources available for those seeking treatment or support.

Teachers and students

The group also took a national approach to introduce mental health curricula specific to schizophrenia into existing health courses in schools. After pilot testing the instructional materials in several different regions, the Local Action Group is currently working to integrate the curricula into the national educational system.

Employers

Cities and communities in which Local Action Groups have been created have established programmes for sheltered employment. Those living with schizophrenia are employed in jobs at a hotel coffee-bar. The hotel project is the model for setting up other 'social firms' projects in Poland.

Church and clergy

The population of Poland is roughly 95% Catholic (75% consider themselves to be 'practising' Catholics). The Local Action Group met with the national organization of the episcopate, which agreed to an educational programme for members of the clergy.

In addition to seminars conducted with the joint cooperation of psychiatrists and the clergy, clerics and monks of the Catholic Church have sponsored fund-raising activities to assist in housing for people with schizophrenia. To date, progress in this area has been slow given complexities and approval processes within the institution of the Church.

A Day of Solidarity

In an effort to further unify efforts on a national level, the group has worked to establish September 15 as 'Day of Solidarity with People Suffering from Schizophrenia'. As noted earlier, the event in 2002 was held in 16 towns and cities. In 2003, this network had expanded to smaller villages as well and totalled 32 communities.

Across the country, mayors of cities and villages, bishops and other clergy, members of the press, and representatives from various NGOs stepped through doorways erected in public squares to show their solidarity for those living with schizophrenia. Cultural events held in many of these locations were broadcast on television.

As a result of this national effort, Polish television produced an educational programme with the active participation of individuals living with schizophrenia.

Overall, the Local Action Group has also presented anti-stigma activities as part of cultural events:

- from 2001 to 2003, more than 10 exhibitions and poetry readings were presented by people living with the illness;
- in 2001, the City of Lodz hosted a theatre festival organized by those with mental illness;

A special focus on youth

Based on the research conducted with young Poles in 2003, and on the fact that first symptoms typically appear in late adolescence and young adulthood, the Local Action Group in programme decided to extend an already successful effort and focus on this younger population.

The 14th of September, the day before the 'Open the Door' Day of Solidarity, was set aside for young people. Workshops were held with a variety of young people, including individuals living with schizophrenia, to educate on the challenges of mental illness but also to celebrate creativity and art with musical and theatrical events. The group promoted their theme 'every one hurts in a different way' across the country.

The largest paper in Poland, *Gazeta Wyborcsa*, is supporting the programme as well. It actively promotes an effort to raise educational standards in the schools to include information on mental health.

The group continues to build on this national interest and awareness, and is planning events throughout the year focused on younger audiences.

- following a screening of *A Beautiful Mind*, a lecture and discussion about schizophrenia with secondary school pupils and students of psychology, medicine and rehabilitation.

A programme called 'Together in Art and Life' has been developed to promote the creative expression of those living with mental illness. The group supports art therapy, organizes exhibitions, auctions, art workshops, courses and conferences as well as fosters relationships with professional artists.

Conclusion

The national effort in Poland continues as of this writing. In 2004, the group held the third National Day of Solidarity with People Suffering from Schizophrenia on 12 September. In Kraków, an exhibition entitled 'Art Against Stigma' was held in the National Museum. A 'Poetry Night' was held in the Slowacki Theatre. During that event the Polish actress Anna Dymna read the poems written by people with schizophrenia and by others, such as Emily Dickinson and Friedrich Holderlin.

Again, the symbolic door was featured in town centres through which individuals step to sign a petition of solidarity.

Compared to other initiatives in the WPA Global Programme, Poland differs in three notable ways:

- Coordination from a central organizing group extending outward, in collaboration, with regional groups, as opposed to regional activities developed independently and reporting back.
- The creation of a high-profile 'National Day of Solidarity' which drew significant attention of the media and generated camaraderie among groups who were geographically distant but working on a common event.
- Its collaboration with religious clergy on the local and national level.

For more information on the Global Programme in Poland, please contact

- Anna Bielánska (Coordinator)
  Day Treatment Centre
  Department of Psychiatry of Jagiellonian University
  31-115 Kraków, Sikorskiego 2/8 Poland
  Phone/Fax: (+48-12) 422 5674
  E-mail: bielania@su.krakow.pl

- Andrzej Cechnicki (Advisor)
  Day Treatment Centre
  Collegium Medicum, Jagiellonian University
  31-115 Kraków, Sikorskiego 2/8 Poland
  Phone: (+48-12) 633 9647
  Fax: (+48-12) 422 5674
  E-mail: mzcechni@cyf-kr.edu.pl

BIBLIOGRAPHY – POLAND

Chadzynska, M., Spiridonow, K., Kasperek, B. and Meder, J. (2003). [Quality of life of schizophrenic patients and their caregivers – comparison.] [Polish] Porownanie jakosci zycia osob chorych na schizofrenie i ich opiekunow. *Psychiatria Polska*, **37**(6), 1025–1036.

Dabrowski, S. (1998). [Specialist community social services as a form of community social support.] [Polish] Specjalistyczne uslugi opiekuncze jako forma oparcia spolecznego. *Psychiatria Polska*, **32**(4), 443–451.

Kucharska-Pietura, K., Grzywa, A. and Debowska, G. (1998). [Attitudes of Polish and British high school students towards the mentally ill and their beliefs in the causes of mental illness.] [Polish] Postawy licealistow z Polski i Wielkiej Brytanii wobec osob psychicznie chorych i ich przekonania na temat etiologii chorob psychicznych. *Psychiatria Polska*, **32**(6), 711–722.

Prot-Herczynska, K. (1998). [The study of the costs of schizophrenia.] [Polish] Badanie kosztow schizofrenii. *Psychiatria Polska*, **32**(3), 307–318.

Wojciechowska, A., Walczewski, K. and Cechnicki, A. (2001). [Correlations between some features of social networks and treatment outcome in patients with schizophrenia three years after initial hospitalization.] [Polish] Zaleznosci miedzy wlasciwosciami sieci spolecznej a wynikami leczenia chorych na schizofrenie w trzy lata od pierwszej hospitalizacji. *Psychiatria Polska*, **35**(1), 21–32.

10

Japan

In 2002, the Japanese Society of Psychiatry and Neurology (JSPN) and the national family organization, Zenkaren, succeeded in changing the name of 'schizophrenia' in order to diminish its stigmatizing effect. The event was unprecedented. There is no other example of a joint effort by psychiatrists and family members to change the name of an illness to reduce the stigma associated with it.

The change of the term 'schizophrenia' has a different significance in Japan from what it might have in most other countries. In 1937, the terminology committee of JSPN translated the term schizophrenia into 精神分裂病, seishin-bunretsu-byo, and reported it as new name of Kraepelin's dementia praecox (i.e. schizophrenia = Dementia praecox). At the time, the concept of schizophrenia was almost identical to dementia praecox and effective medications were unavailable. They believed 精神分裂病, seishin-bunretsu-byo, to be untreatable with no chance for recovery and with progressive deterioration. In addition, because 精神分裂病, seishin-bunretsu-byo literally means 'split mind', Eugen Bleuler's attempt to describe the individual as 'cut off from' or 'dissociated from' affect became in the translation a description of an individual cut-off from the essence of his or her humanity. As one individual living schizophrenia put it speaking at the World Psychiatric Association (WPA) Congress in 1998, 'This term tells me I am cut off from my soul'.

Earlier, we described attempts to disrupt the vicious cycle of stigmatization with interventions at different points on the cycle. In the case of efforts in Japan, by disrupting the stigma of the name itself, the Japanese hope to reduce the downstream social consequences of the labelling.

In 1993, Zenkaren, the National Federation of Families with Mental Illness, had made a formal request to the JSPN to change the Japanese term for schizophrenia. The JSPN organized a Committee on Concepts and Terminology of Mental Disorders to look into the problem.

In 1998, the JSPN began working with the WPA Global Programme against Stigma and Discrimination because of Schizophrenia. The efforts to possibly change the terminology – and change the associated stigma – were of considerable interest to the global effort. If effective, a similar change might be promoted in other countries using translations or descriptions of mental illness. An announcement of that collaboration was made at the World Congress of Psychiatry in Hamburg, Germany.

Research regarding the term was conducted with psychiatrists, people with schizophrenia and their family members. The committee narrowed the field to three options in 2001:

- The rendering of the word 'schizophrenia' into katakana, a symbol system to phonetically designate words, generally of foreign origin – *sukizofurenia*.
- Togo-shiccho-sho, 統合失調症, meaning 'thought integration disorder'.
- 'Kraepelin–Bleuler Disease' referring to Emil Kraepelin and Eugen Bleuler, two of the psychiatrists chiefly responsible for the systematic diagnosis of the illness and its course.

In 2001, in an interview with a Japanese newspaper, Professor Mitsumoto Sato, Chairman of the Committee, discussed the renaming of schizophrenia and the alternatives being considered. Among those living with the illness, he reported, one-third were accepting of the old name, one-third would have used the foreign name, *sukizofurenia*; and one-third preferred the use of the new word. After a series of surveys of JSPN council members and the Zenkaren members, a public hearing was held. In February 2002, based upon responses from all groups, the Board of JSPN selected a term and proposed it to the general assembly of JSPN in August 2002. Then, the decision to use 統合失調症, Togo-shiccho-sho, was announced at the WPA Congress in 2002 in Yokohama, Japan. Following this announcement, the Ministry of Health, Labour and Welfare immediately approved the use of the new name in every public document relating to the Mental Health and Welfare Act and for medical fee invoicing.

Notices were also sent out to all department heads in Japan's 12 major cities and all local governments. Releases to the media and press requested that they no longer use the older term.

Follow-up research on effectiveness

To measure the effectiveness of the diffusion of the new term, the Japanese government supported five studies.

Study 1: Japanese psychiatrists

Many Japanese psychiatrists are reluctant to tell their patients what their diagnosis is. This reluctance is even sharper in the case of 'schizophrenia' than with other diagnoses. The first study was conducted after the introduction of the new term and assessed all 8517 psychiatrists of the JSPN. A questionnaire and postage-paid reply were sent to the association list. Researchers received 4027 responses (47.3%). The research found:

- The new and old names were being used together.
- The older the doctor, the more negative the attitude towards informing the patient of the diagnosis or using the new name; compared to those in outpatient clinics, psychiatrists affiliated with university and psychiatric hospitals were more likely to use the new term and inform patients of the diagnosis.
- Results varied in different regions of the country in terms of psychiatrists tendency to inform the consumer or family members.

A study was also conducted of the frequency of its use in official documents – as required by the Mental Health and Welfare Act – and for medical fee invoicing. In the period from April 2002 to January 2003, 2812 documents in the Miyagi Prefecture were examined. By December 2002, use of the new name had increased to 76%. A second survey of 61 Prefectures in Japan found the term used an average of 78% of the time (Sato *et al.*, 2004).

Study 2: Individuals diagnosed with schizophrenia

Ten questionnaires were sent to all 512 rehabilitation facilities. These question-naires were forwarded to those diagnosed with schizophrenia and 2500 (48.8%) responded. Among the results gathered from this group:

- 72% of the respondents said they had been treated for schizophrenia for more than 5 years;
- 51% regularly visit the rehabilitation facility but live with parents or friends;
- the majority never discuss the illness except with their doctors;
- while many respondents knew of the new term, few used it to refer to themselves.

Study 3: Family members

The third study examined the attitudes of relatives regarding the name change. Questionnaires were sent to members of the Zenkaren Family Association and 987 (39.5%) responded.

Seventy-seven per cent reported feeling positive about the change of the term. Outside of the local medical administrative office, family members felt that the local community was not supportive of the family or the individual living with schizophrenia.

Study 4: General public/college students

The fourth study examined community attitudes about the change of the termin-ology and general attitudes regarding those with the illness. A survey was conducted among two groups of students at Keio University.

Both groups watched the movie, *A Beautiful Mind*, the story of Nobel Prize winning mathematician and consumer, John Nash. The first group of 133 students were given a pre-test using the older, traditional term. The second group was given a questionnaire using the new name.

The two groups showed marked differences in their responses:

- before watching the film, those given the newer term reported a lower negative image of the term than those in the group using the traditional term;
- after viewing the movie, the new name had a further positive image;
- the effect upon attitudes after viewing the movie was lower among those using the older term;
- the group given the older term showed improved attitudes regarding social disadvantages after viewing the film;
- both groups showed improved attitudes towards the efficacy of treatment after viewing the film.

Study 5: Psychiatric professionals in universities

A survey was conducted among psychiatric professors teaching undergraduate and postgraduate students. Questionnaires with postage-paid replies were sent to all 84 national psychiatric professors regarding their attitudes towards teaching students about the new term. Roughly 52% (44 professors) responded.

To the question 'How do you educate postgraduates on informing patients about schizophrenia?' a majority advised their students to use discretion.

When asked 'How often do you use the traditional term for schizophrenia?', respondents said they used the term in clinical and educational situations more often than in written documents. When asked 'How often do you use the new term?' they reported using it more often with families and in educational situations.

Overall, the respondents said they used both terms in educational settings, but not in documentation.

Guidelines for the future

Overall, one major challenge in the transition to the new term is that those who have lived in the community in the past have received pensions of 83,000 yen per month from the government for the diagnosis of 'severe schizophrenia'. Individuals living with schizophrenia and their families have expressed concern that changing the diagnosis may lead to a suspension of government funding.

The Japanese Local Action Group is currently investigating ways to help, make the transition in the terminology without jeopardizing benefits.

In addition, the group has recommended guidelines for describing the illness to various target audiences. These guidelines call for using the new term without explaining it in relation to the older term. Guidelines are being developed for: medical specialists, people living with the illness and family members, and the general public including journalists and the media.

In 2004, the Local Action Group began examining ways to further involve psychiatric professors in the active dissemination of the new term. Because of their distance from the clinical setting and influence on students at both the under- and postgraduate levels, the Local Action Group sees this as an especially important initiative.

Through their continued efforts at all levels – from the individual consumer to society, from teacher to student – the Japanese Local Action Group is working to implement the new term and in turn, achieve a reduction in stigma and prejudice. Understanding that this second goal would require more than a word change, they have pursued additional anti-stigma interventions.

Working in the community

In 2000, the JSPN formed an *ad-hoc* committee to develop and implement an anti-stigma programme in cooperation with the WPA global initiatives. After several initial planning meetings, the group expanded its membership to include politicians from the Diet, patient activists and representatives from family associations.

Space does not allow us to explore all of the unique aspects of psychiatry as it is practiced in Japan. Three features are important, however, in understanding the aspects of the interventions undertaken:

- individuals living with schizophrenia spend on average much longer periods in institutions than in other industrialized countries;
- social stigma for the individual and the family in the community is especially high;
- polypharmacy and the overall consumption of anti-psychotics is one of the highest per capita in the world.

Three sites were selected for initial pilot testing of the programme in Japan: Tokachi (in the northern Prefecture), Sendai (in the Miyagi Prefecture) and Okayama (west of Tokyo). Groups were then organized in these cities and included: physicians, social workers and psychologists as well as individuals living with schizophrenia and family members. With its infrastructure in place, the national initiative held a public forum on 27 August 2002 at the WPA World Congress in Yokohama.

Each region has developed interventions based on its own community profile. Yet all data has been presented to the central group affiliated with the JSPN.

Tokachi

The northern island of Hokkaido has a total population of 5,702,000 yet the Prefecture of Tokachi alone is geographically 5 times the size of metropolitan Tokyo. Obihiro, the capital of Tokachi, has a population of 171,557.

The Local Action Group assembled there consisted of 11 members, actively involving people living with schizophrenia in research design and programme preparation. The group selected high school students as the first target for their intervention.

Pre- and post-tests were conducted in two high schools. Of the 303 students, 174 were male and 129 were female. The group used the Alberta questionnaire translated into Japanese with slight modifications.

In one class a member of a consumer advocacy group shared his own experiences of schizophrenia and the associated stigma. In the second class, a psychiatrist presented a medical explanation of schizophrenia, which included information on the ratio of in- and outpatients, the number of psychiatric beds, comparison of the average length of hospitalization between Japan and other countries.

Pre- and post-test results indicated that students rated the time spent with the person diagnosed with schizophrenia more effective than the time with the psychiatrist. Measurements of knowledge and attitudes bore out this claim.

In August 2003, a focus group intervention indicated that individuals diagnosed with schizophrenia find family members, medical staff, employers and co-workers among the most stigmatizing groups.

Based on these finding, the group developed additional interventions. The first of these were events and meetings at which people with schizophrenia and their families meet with other families as well. These individuals are encouraged to share their experiences and discuss strategies for developing the communal support that may be lacking in their neighbourhoods.

To address the issues surrounding challenges to employment, the group has made contact with labour unions. The plan is to present educational programmes, which include interactive games and group discussions with members of these unions to decrease the stigma associated with schizophrenia and enlist the support of unions for those living with the illness.

Sendai

The city of Sendai, located in the northeast of the central island of Japan, has a population of 1,024,80. It is the capital of the Miyagi prefecture.

In 1982, the Japanese government introduced statutory home help service for individuals with physical disabilities. In 1999, an amendment of the Mental Health and Welfare Act endorsed home help services for individuals living with mental illness. Research by Zenkaren found that a significant number of home-helpers expressed anxiety about working with individuals with mental illness (Maruyama *et al.*, 2001.)

To change this, two different interventions were conducted. In the first, home helpers were segmented into discussion groups based upon the number of patients in their charge. The groups discussed:

1 the kinds of stigma and discrimination, which mentally ill patients face;
2 the causes of this stigma and discrimination;
3 what is needed to reduce that stigma.

Following this discussion, a psychiatrist presented a lecture on the prevalence, symptoms, course, prognosis, cause, treatment and rehabilitation of the illness.

In the second intervention session, the lecture from the psychiatrist was followed by a discussion that included individuals living with schizophrenia, who dealt with the topics of stigma and discrimination discussed in the first session.

Research was conducted in two districts in Sendai with 85 home helpers participating. Ninety-seven did not participate. Overall, in this group, interactions with people living with schizophrenia significantly improved attitudes. Furthermore, when research was compared between participants (59 questionnaires completed) and non-participants (43 of whom agreed to complete the questionnaires), participants showing a marked increase in knowledge and decrease in social distance when compared with non-participants.

Another significant outcome of this intervention is that the people with schizophrenia, who participated in the intervention described above, continued meeting and established the first self-help group for mental illness in that district.

Okayama

Okayama Prefecture is located in the western portion of the central island of Japan. The population of Okayama City is 626,642, roughly one-third of the population of the overall Prefecture.

The Local Action Group, led by Dr Kenzo Fujita, consists of nine professionals, family members and individuals living with the schizophrenia. The educational format used was similar to that in both Tokachi and Sendai; however, the target group chosen was different.

Local welfare commissioners are retired and elderly members of the community charged with assisting neighbours in receiving welfare services they may require. Given the tendency for more elderly men and women to display greater social distance towards those with mental illness, this was viewed as a particularly challenging target group.

A total of 234 local welfare commissioners participated in the research. They were divided into three groups of 78 each. The first group was given conventional training of a lecture by a psychiatrist. The second group received a similar lecture which was then followed by a 'get-acquainted' session involving five-to-seven commissioners, one or two mental health professionals, and two or three individuals living with schizophrenia.

Results from Okayama reinforce the importance of personal contact with an individual living with mental illness in overcoming stereotypes and stigma. Following this intervention, patient's advocates were recruited publicly and they continue to assist in ongoing anti-stigma efforts with this target audience.

Moving forward

The finding of the three Japanese Local Action Groups confirmed long-standing research from other countries on the effectiveness of personal contact in improving attitudes towards those with mental illness. More important, however, is the momentum generated through the coordination of the three centres.

In 2003, a Local Action Group was established in Ichikawa. The groups consist of the president of the district association for medical doctors, a staff member of the health centre, a city hall officer, a journalist, a consumer and a family member.

The group has conducted five focus groups to identify sources of stigma and discrimination which has mirrored findings from Tokachi.

The Local Action Groups are also meeting regularly with members of the Diet to make them more aware of legislation and government action that can reduce stigma and discrimination, and provide greater support for those living with mental illness.

The web site, www.openthedoors.com, has also been translated into Japanese and is routinely updated with information for those living with schizophrenia, their families and professionals: http://www.openthedoors.com/japanese/index.html.

For more information on the Global Programme in Japan, please contact

- Mitsumoto Sato (Coordinator)
  Tohoku Fukushi University
  1-8-1 Kunimi, Aoba-ku Sendai, Miyagi 981-8522, Japan
  E-mail: mitsu@tfu-mail.tfu.ac.jp
- Yuki Nishimura
  Health Center, Keio University

4-1-1 Hiyoshi, Kohokuku, Yokohama, Kanagawa 223-8521, Japan
E-mail: ynishi@hc.cc.keio.ac.jp
• Masaaki Nishio
Department of Psychiatric Rehabilitation
National Institute of Mental Health
Konodai 1-7-3, Echikawa, Chiba, Japan
E-mail: nishio@ncnp-k.go.jp

REFERENCES – JAPAN

Sato, M., *et al.* (2004). Correction of stigma against schizophrenia by renewing the name and disease concept of schizophrenia in Japan. [Japanese]. *Journal of Comprehensive Welfare*, **2**, 17–33.

Maruyama, Y., Taira, N., Mita, Y. and Oshima, I. (2001). The role of people with mental disorders to reduce discrimination and stigma. *Society for Disability Studies 2001 Conference Proceedings*, p 33–37.

BIBLIOGRAPHY – JAPAN

Anzai, N., Yoneda, S., Kumagai, N., Nakamura, Y., Ikebuchi, E. and Liberman, R.P. (2002). Training persons with schizophrenia in illness self-management: a randomized controlled trial in Japan. *Psychiatric Services*, **53**(5), 545–547.

Chong, M.-Y., Tan, C.H., Fujii, S., Uang, S.-Y., Ungvari, F.S., Si, T., Chung, E.K., Sim, K., Tsang, H.-Y. and Shinfuku, N. (2004). Antipsychotic drug prescription for schizophrenia in East Asia: rational for change. *Psychiatry and Clinical Neurosciences*, **58**, 61–67.

Hershey, L. (2001). Researchers find limited support for independence in japan: people with physical and mental disabilities face two distinct sets of obstacles. *Disability World*, Issue no. 9.

Ito, T. (2004). [Medical, practical and sociocultural significance in changing the disease name for schizophrenia in Japan.] [Japanese] *Seishin Shinkeigaku Zasshi – Psychiatria et Neurologia Japonica*, **106**(3), 321–325.

Nakane, A. (2004). [Influence of changing the disease name for schizophrenia on Japanese patients' quality of life.] [Japanese] *Seishin Shinkeigaku Zasshi – Psychiatria et Neurologia Japonica*, **106**(3), 326–331.

Ono, H. and Nishimura, Y. (2004). [Change in the disease name for schizophrenia in Japan and its effect on informed consent given by physicians.] [Japanese] *Seishin Shinkeigaku Zasshi – Psychiatria et Neurologia Japonica*, **106**(3), 313–316.

Pearson, N.O. (2004). Suicides in Japan hit record high in 2003. *The Washington Post*, The Associated Press.

Sato, M. (2004). [Changing the disease name for schizophrenia in Japan.] [Japanese] *Seishin Shinkeigaku Zasshi – Psychiatria et Neurologia Japonica*, **106**(3), 311–312.

Takagi, S. (2004). [Process and future tasks in changing the disease name for schizophrenia in Japan.] [Japanese] *Seishin Shinkeigaku Zasshi – Psychiatria et Neurologia Japonica*, **106**(3), 332–334.

Takei, N., Inagaki, A., and JPSS-2 research group. (2002). Polypharmacy for psychiatric treatments in Japan. *The Lancet*, **360**, p 647.

Uranaka, T. (2000). Local autonomy put to test by new nursing care program. *The Japan Times*. The Japan Times Ltd.

Yamakado, T. (2004). [Influence of changing the disease name for schizophrenia on clinical practice of psychiatry in community psychiatric hospitals in Japan.] [Japanese] *Seishin Shinkeigaku Zasshi – Psychiatria et Neurologia Japonica*, **106**(3), 317–320.

Phase IV

11

Slovakia

'The boss is the patient.' It is a phrase that Pětr Nawka uses in his talks on fighting the stigma and discrimination because of schizophrenia. 'Real reform,' he adds, 'arises from the needs of the patient.' *The Boss is the Patient* has also become the title of a film developed in a collaboration between Dr Nawka and Irsinnig Menschlich (Madly Human), the consumer activist group in Leipzig, Germany.

Prior to organizing the Local Action Group in Slovakia with Charlene Reiss, Dr Nawka had already begun to develop innovative ways of engaging individuals living with schizophrenia in confronting the self-stigma that can accompany the experience of schizophrenia. In Slovakia, he introduced the concept of *stigma-journaling*, having individuals record their experiences of stigma. The video project in Leipzig was conducted in the same spirit of empowering people living with the illness, using the video camera as a kind of electronic journal to record thoughts, ideas and experiences.

A centrepiece of Dr Nawka's presentation and approach is his reliance upon a 'tetralogue model' in addressing issues related to treatment of psychiatric illnesses. The four components of this model are individuals living with schizophrenia, professionals, family members and caregivers, and society. Only by addressing the needs of all four constituencies in the 'conversation,' Nawka maintains, will effective treatment be possible. Opposition from any one area – a lack of funding, insufficient support from physicians or family, or an absence of active involvement from the individual living with the illness themselves can doom the most well-intentioned effort. As Dr Nawka puts it: 'consumers, their relatives and professionals coming together to form a trialogue, makes the possibility of bringing society into tetralogue easier – demonstrating the ability of the trialogue's participants to overcome self-stigma and mutual stigma as well.'

Starting in Michalovce

The city of Michalovce, located in Eastern Slovakia, has a population of 40,000. The first meeting of the Local Action Group included the President of the

National Organization of Consumers' Organizations, the President of the National Organization of Relatives, one psychiatrist and two non-medical volunteers.

One of the first initiatives of the Local Action Group in January 2001 was a survey of individuals living with schizophrenia, families, and mental health professionals in Michalovce, regarding their personal experiences of stigma and discrimination. Based on these results, the group selected their initial target audiences:

- general and mental health care professionals;
- families;
- high school students and teachers;
- general public through a focus on journalists and other members of the media.

The group agreed upon the name *Otvorme dvere – otvorme srdcia* (ODOS) (Open the Doors, Open your Hearts). They established the group as a new Non-Governmental Organization (NGO) to address the goals of the World Psychiatric Association (WPA) global programme for Slovakia and determined the need to bring on new partners. ODOS is now a member of the Slovak League for Mental Health. With the assistance of Eli Lilly and the League of Mental Health, the group was able to hire a director and secretariat for the program and successfully expand their efforts to the country's capital of Bratislava.

The four goals of the Local Action Group have been:

- to reintegrate people with mental illness back into society;
- to protect the human rights of people with mental illness;
- to achieve parity between the treatment of physical and mental illnesses in Slovakia;
- to promote the mental health of society as a whole.

Key to the group's mission is an effort to help individuals living with the illness to overcome self-stigma and become more actively involved in their own treatment. For example, members of the Patients' Advocates Club visit individuals during hospitalization to address the questions and fears they may have.

Working with the Slovak League of Mental Health, the Local Action Group has been successful in keeping the issue of stigma as a focus of professional conferences. Stigma has also become a subject of discussion and action with patient advocacy groups and events on Mental Health Day.

ODOS has also formed a partnership with the Slovak Association of Relatives, Opora. In cooperation with the European Federation of Associations of Families of Mentally Ill People (EUFAMI), an educational project was developed for people living with the illness, family members and medical professionals. The programme trains educators who will work in different regions of the country.

In a further attempt to educate health care professionals, the Local Action Group used the focus group method to discuss coercive measures in treatment. Based on the findings from this study, ODOS is bringing researchers and clinicians together with individuals living with schizophrenia, relatives, mental health advocates, and legal experts to assess the issue of coercion in psychiatric admission and treatment. By examining those areas where consumers' rights may have been violated, the group will develop recommendations for reforming the process and avoiding the negative therapeutic effects of the process itself.

Changing, not fighting, the system

In 2003, the Local Action Group undertook a 3-year pilot project entitled 'Transformation to an Integrated System of Mental Healthcare' in partnership with the Association for Mental Health Integra. Professionals from all 15 major Slovak institutions working directly (and indirectly) with mental health are involved. The Ministry of Health has assigned six advisors to the project – with the goal of creating a new system of care in the field of social medicine. The group is currently preparing legislation for long-term care, thus integrating care for people with severe mental disorders with general health and social care. In addition, the pilot project objectives include establishing eight sites for sheltered living, ten sites for active employment, thirty rehabilitation centres and a case management team.

In April 2003, a tea house was opened in the centre of Michalovce as one of the first pilot sites for employment. In addition to empowering people living with schizophrenia with economic opportunities, the tea house also provides opportunities for the public to interact with the consumers to overcome prejudices and misconceptions, and potentially to develop a deeper social network.

A case management team was formed in March 2003. Since that time, they have developed a programme to support people with schizophrenia to live in the community. The team works in close cooperation with the health and social services in the region and, together with the consumers, develops individual therapeutic and rehabilitation plans.

Working with and through the media

If one axis of the programme has been to further empower individuals living with schizophrenia and reduce self-stigma, the second axis is an effort to reach the general public by working through the media. As mentioned earlier, Dr Nawka has worked closely with the consumer organization Irrsinnig Menschlich from Leipzig, Germany.

From July 2002 through May 2003, Irrsinnig Menschlich worked with the Club of People with Schizophrenia in Slovakia and a local television station. Club members from Slovakia and consumers from Leipzig received training in film-making, learning narrative and technical skills to best communicate their stories.

The workshop was entitled 'Against the Images in our Heads.' Together the group wrote, directed and produced the feature film, *The Boss is the Patient* and debuted the film at the *Second International Conference on Stigma and Discrimination because of Schizophrenia* held in Kingston, Canada in October 2003. On 19 March 2004, the film aired on the European television channel, ARTE, as part of an evening devoted to the subject of schizophrenia.

From the first meeting of the NGO, ODOS, the Local Action Group has been working to develop an ongoing dialogue with the media. Media contact lists prepared for journalists have led to interviews with individuals living with schizophrenia, relatives, and health care professionals appearing in magazines and newspapers, as well as on national and local television. A three-page article on people living with schizophrenia appeared in Slovakia's most popular weekly magazine with a circulation of more than 100,000. The article included interviews with, and photographs of, individuals living with the illness and their families.

The network of people living with schizophrenia, family members and mental health professionals has been invaluable for ensuring stigma remains a topic presented at professional conferences, schools, and the annual national meeting of Slovak mental health users. Members of the Local Action Group were also invited by the Slovak Humanitarian Council to speak with the president of the Slovak Republic about stigma and other mental health issues. This meeting received extensive coverage in the media and has helped publicize the national anti-stigma movement.

ODOS established a local club in Michalovce for people living with schizophrenia that focuses on educating the public and the media. Club members meet weekly to discuss schizophrenia and stigma. They also receive training in public speaking and some individuals now speak regularly to high school students about mental health issues.

Conclusion

What is the tipping point of a programme? When can it move from a local initiative in a city of 40,000 to a national campaign with an office in the country's capital city? Clearly the dedication of Pĕtr Nawka is one important element. But a programme might just as likely become bogged down in local details if the lead organizer becomes the lone spokesperson or face to the media.

Two elements have been essential in the national – indeed, international – reach of the work in Slovakia: alliances and empowerment of those living with schizophrenia. Political alliances have been formed through the Slovak League of Mental Health and subsequently with the Slovak Humanitarian Council. Greater empowerment has come through training programmes in public speaking and the establishment of a special Club of People with Schizophrenia.

For more information on the Global Programme in Slovakia, please contact

- Pĕtr Nawka (Coordinator)
  Psychiatric Hospital
  A. Hrehovčika 1
  SK-07101 Michalovce, Slovakia
  Phone: (+42-15) 66431715
  Fax: (+42-15) 66884822
  E-mail: nawka@pnmi.sk

REFERENCES – SLOVAKIA

Nawka, P. and Reiss, C.M. (2002). Integrating people who are stigmatized: the tetralogue model. *World Psychiatry*, **16**(1), 1.

Nawka, P., Reiss, C.M. and Dolobac, L. (2002). The antistigma action programme in Slovakia: a catalyst to integration. *European Psychiatry*, **17**(0), 81.

12

Turkey

In 2003, a study of public attitudes in rural Turkey towards those living with schizophrenia revealed that half of the 208 adults in a village near Manisa believe that persons with schizophrenia are aggressive and should not be free in the community. Manisa is 30 km North-east of Izmir on the Aegean coast. An even greater number said they would be irritated knowing that a neighbour had schizophrenia (61.5%). A similar number (61.1%) said that they would not rent their home to a person with schizophrenia and 85.6% said they would not marry someone with schizophrenia.

At the same time this study was being conducted, Dr Alp Üçok, head of the Local Action Group in Istanbul, was conducting another survey on the attitudes of psychiatrists towards those diagnosed with schizophrenia. Questionnaires were distributed to 100 members of the Schizophrenia Section of the Psychiatric Association of Turkey. Sixty psychiatrists (40 men and 20 women) from five cities responded. Twenty-three of the respondents worked in a university hospital, 22 in a general state hospital and 15 in a psychiatric hospital. The mean age of the psychiatrists was 37 and the mean duration of practice in psychiatry was 9.8 years.

While the sample size may at first seem small, it represents 5% of all psychiatrists (including residents) in Turkey. World Health Organization (WHO) statistics currently place the number of psychiatrists in Turkey at 1 per 100,000.[1]

Forty-two per cent of the psychiatrists surveyed responded that they never informed patients of the diagnosis of schizophrenia. Roughly 17% said they always informed patients and 40.7% said they did so on a case-by-case basis.

Among the most common reasons given was that patients and family members could not understand the meaning of schizophrenia (32.6%). (This in contrast to the study by Taskin *et al.*, which found that respondents in the rural villages claim to understand the term 'schizophrenia'.) They also believed patients and/or family members would drop out of treatment (28.3%) or become demoralized (13.5%) if

---

[1] This compared to 16 per 100,000 in the US.

they learned the diagnosis. Slightly more than half (55.2%) expressed discomfort when meeting a patient with schizophrenia at a social event.

Can an anti-stigma campaign succeed against such strong social stigma when the psychiatric community itself holds such negative attitudes? A third study from Turkey published in 2003, found that the attitudes of non-psychiatric physicians towards the mentally ill were worse than those of the hospital staff in an university hospital.

Building a programme and a non-governmental organization

Based on earlier examples of work at other World Psychiatric Association (WPA) sites, in April and May 2000, Dr Üçok, conducted interviews with individuals living with schizophrenia and family members as to the challenges of stigma and discrimination they perceived. At the same time, a study was conducted to establish whether the stigma related to mental disorders was specific to schizophrenia. The group found stigma extended beyond schizophrenia.

Given the level of stigma in both the general public and medical community, the Local Action Group knew the importance of bringing together different constituencies to achieve the greatest reach. Working in close collaboration with the Psychiatric Association of Turkey and the Association of Family Physicians and General Practitioners, the Local Action Group assisted in the creation of the first Non-Governmental Organization (NGO) dedicated to mental health in Turkey – 'Association of Friends for Schizophrenia'. The announcement of this group coincided with the launch in January 2001 of the Open the Doors programme in Istanbul.

Two university clinics in Istanbul and Marmara leant their support to the programme. At Istanbul's Bilgi University, the Media Department agreed to provide logistical support to help disseminate programme communications.

Efforts in 2001 focused on metropolitan Istanbul. The initial target audiences chosen were general practitioners (GPs), medical students, school counsellors and teachers, journalists, and the general public.

In 2002, these initiatives were broadened to the capital of Ankara, Izmir to the southwest and Erzurum in Eastern Anatolia.

General practitioners

Given the relatively low number of psychiatrists per capita and the negative attitudes uncovered by the research, the Local Action Group has focused much of its efforts on general practitioners.

Copies of Volume II of the WPA materials, dealing with the latest scientific information on schizophrenia and its treatment, were translated into Turkish and distributed to each medical centre in Istanbul. Information packets on early diagnosis were developed specifically for GPs. These kits included handouts of a slide presentation, a chart for prodromal symptoms and a chart on daily doses of antipsychotics in maintenance of schizophrenia. Three hundred were distributed on the European side of Istanbul and 200 were distributed to the Eastern, Asian community.

During the initial phases of the programme, from 2001 to well into 2002, the group held weekly meetings with GPs and family physicians. In 2003, a series of four larger meetings were held in Istanbul and Ankara.

Each meeting began with a 45-min presentation on schizophrenia – symptoms of the illness, the public health burden, the GP's role in its diagnosis and treatment. The presentation was followed by an interactive session using more case-related questions. Participants are encouraged to provide insights and feedback for both the presentation and on the anti-stigma programme.

Efforts continued with psychiatrists as well. The central theme of the Twelfth National Congress on Social Psychiatry was 'Stigma and Mental Health'. More than 10 panel discussions and conference presentations focused on the reasons for and effect of stigma related to mental illness. Professor Julian Leff, chairman of the Reintegration Committee of the WPA Global Programme, presented an overview of the stigma related to schizophrenia around the world.

In April 2003, at the Spring Symposia of the Psychiatric Association of Turkey, the Local Action Group organized a panel discussion entitled: 'Stigma and Schizophrenia: What More Can We Be Doing?' A consumer and a family member were among the speakers at the symposium sharing their experiences with professionals.

Finally, interactive workshops on stigma have been prepared for sixth year medical students. These workshops are presented to those in psychiatry rotations at Marmara and Istanbul University. A course entitled: 'The Attitudes of Society and Doctors Toward Mental Illness' has been part of the curriculum at Istanbul Faculty of Medicine. Since 1999, more than 400 students have attended the course.

Working with the general public

Like the initiative underway in Poland, the Local Action Group in Turkey has organized a public event to increase public awareness and build community among people living with schizophrenia, family members and medical professionals. The event, called Schizophrenia Walk, was begun in May 2001 in Istanbul. The fourth Schizophrenia Walk was held on 18 September 2004.

Each year, the group has seen a significant increase in media coverage in magazines, newspapers and on televisions. The most notable rise in media interest came after a press conference held during the third annual event in 2003. Working with the NGO, Association of Friends for Schizophrenia, the group distributed information brochures as well as caps and keyholders imprinted with the logo and motto of the family association.

One result of the media interest has been a pair of meetings held with journalists in October 2002 and April 2003. Members of the Association of Health Reporters attended both meetings. At these meetings, a family member recounted her experiences with stigma and professionals provided medical information on schizophrenia and its treatment.

In early 2004, a media kit was developed for journalists. The group is also supporting the dissemination of information on web sites of a consumer association. The programme now has an official journal, entitled *Kapıları Acin* (Open the Doors). It features information regarding on-going activities and contact information.

A film by family members appeared on 10 television stations across Turkey. Six other television programmes – specifically dealing with schizophrenia and the WPA anti-stigma efforts – appeared in May and June 2001.

The Department of Communication of Bilgi University prepared 10 short video clips – containing anti-stigma messages – which aired on national television stations in late 2001. This media effort, in turn, generated more publicity on national radio and television programmes.

Consumer and family members

The NGO, Association of Friends for Schizophrenia, was created in part to address the need of individuals living with schizophrenia and family members for organized support.

The group has helped assemble five informational booklets for individuals living with schizophrenia and family members: 'What is schizophrenia', 'Schizophrenia and the Family', 'Legal Issues', 'Therapy' and 'Course of the Illness'. In addition to distribution to family members, the brochure 'What is Schizophrenia' is used at public meetings and events on stigma. Ten focus groups were conducted to explore the needs of the caregivers in the period of 2001–2002 in Istanbul. A survey on the level of stigmatization by the family members and caregivers is also underway.

High school students and teachers

In March 2002, the Local Action Group began an educational programme to teachers and counsellors in high schools. Members of local action team reached about a 1000 students and 100 teachers in 2002. The following year, a study was completed in two of the main high schools on the Anatolian side of Istanbul. Based on these results, the Local Action Group has developed a curriculum for use in high schools. This programme was put into action in Izmir in 2004. Several meetings were held in high schools: two of these high schools are being evaluated for the outcomes in developing curricula to improve knowledge and attitudes about schizophrenia. Recommendations for this curriculum accompanied a report to the Ministry of Education, evaluating health and psychology class materials.

Conclusion

Both the interventions in high schools and general health care setting were encouraged and faced little opposition. Today, anti-stigma education modules are part of internship training in both Istanbul and Marmara Medical Schools.

When asked to cite the major accomplishment of the programme to date, Dr Üçok discusses the way in which 'psychiatrists and other mental health professionals have become part of the health promotion activities in different regions (Erzurum, Ankara, Urfa, and Izmir). And as a result several studies and research proposals are now focusing specifically on stigmatization because of schizophrenia'.

He also sees a strong, on-going exchange between the Local Action Group and the association, Friends for Schizophrenia. Working together, they continue to broaden the reach of the programme and its message to politicians and the general public.

For more information on the Global Programme in Turkey, please contact:

- Alp Üçok (Coordinator)
  Department of Psychiatry, Istanbul Medical Faculty
  Millet street, 34390 Çapa, Istanbul , Turkey
  Phone: (+49-212) 4142000 31328
  E-mail: alpucok@superonline.com

BIBLIOGRAPHY – TURKEY

Aydin, N., Yigit, A., Inandi, T. and Kirpinar, I. (2003). Attitudes of hospital staff toward mentally ill patients in a teaching hospital, Turkey. *International Journal of Social Psychiatry*, **49**(1), 17–26.

Project Atlas: Country Profile: Turkey. (2002). World Health Organization.

Taskin, E.O., Sen, F.S., Aydemir, O., Demet, M.M., Ozmen, E. and Icelli, I. (2003). Public attitudes to schizophrenia in rural Turkey. *Social Psychiatry and Psychiatric Epidemiology*, **38**(10), 586–592.

Üçok, A., Polat, A., Sartorius, N., Erkoc, S. and Atakli, C. (2004). Attitudes of psychiatrists toward patients with schizophrenia. *Psychiatry and Clinical Neurosciences*, **58**(1), 89–91.

13

Brazil

I want to be bigger than I am now
Maybe with a glimpse of the world gone by
I want to study very, very, very much
And learn more every time

And more: learn with life and other people
And more: live freely
Always be me as well as being somebody
And, when I fall, be able to get up

The poem above was written by Arlindo da Cunha Campello. Entitled 'My ego and the desire', it is based on a poem by Ricardo Reis and was written as part of a Writing Workshop in 2002 as one of the many activities of the Local Action Group's efforts in Brazil.

Establishing the programme

The number of individuals living with schizophrenia in Brazil is estimated at roughly 1.7 million. From 1984 to 1996, the health care system reduced the number of psychiatric beds by 36%. Unfortunately, the development of community-based services, while gradually improving, are grossly underfunded. Most health care services for the mentally ill are provided by the private sector.

The majority of Brazilians have poor access to health care and those who do report a poor quality of care. The human rights of the mentally ill, as well as the under-diagnosis of mental illnesses have yet to be adequately addressed by public health policies and services.

According to Dr Cecília Villares, programme coordinator of the Local Action Group in Brazil: 'For many, prejudice and discrimination constitute an everyday experience. Among the difficulties and obstacles faced, lack of adequate treatment settings, lack of education, poor access to information and lack of legal and social support are some of the major issues related to stigma and discrimination experienced by people diagnosed with schizophrenia and their caregivers'.

In 2000, the WPA Steering Committee began conversations with the Brazilian Psychiatric Association and its then President, Professor Miguel Jorge, regarding the start of an anti-stigma effort in his country. In early 2001, a planning group met in São Paulo to discuss preliminary steps for the development of the programme. The planning group agreed to form two executive committees: the Coordinating Committee and the Local Action Group. The Local Action Group was comprised of nine members that included mental health professionals and a journalist. Each member of the Local Action Group was responsible for helping to coordinate specific interventions.

Targeting two communities

Estimates place the population of the Greater São Paulo metro area at 20 million people, making it the most populous city in the Southern Hemisphere. To implement a programme in an urban centre with the population greater than the country of Chile, the Local Action Group directed its efforts to two communities.

First, the Psychiatric Department of São Paulo Federal University (UNIFESP) already had an established Schizophrenia Programme made up of patients, family members and professionals. The group known as Programa de Esquizofrenia (PROESQ) provides outpatient services within the hospital and has become a centre for graduate and post-graduate training and research on schizophrenia.

Patients from every region of the city as well as outlying districts utilize these services due to their comparatively high quality of care and the multidisciplinary nature of care. The established strengths of PROESQ and its proximity to the University community of students, professors and employees made it an ideal incubator for generating community action and actively involving those living with schizophrenia and their family members.

Second, the UNIFESP also runs the psychiatric services at Pirajussara Hospital, a 200-bed hospital with ten psychiatric beds, a day hospital and outpatient services. The community of the Pirajussara Region within the São Paulo metropolitan region is made up of two neighbouring urban centres, Embú (population: 207,000) and Taboão (population: 198,000). Both areas have a high density of lower income families and served as models for other urban settings in Brazil. A community centre was scheduled to be opened in Pirajussara in 2002 and the group felt that successful interventions in this community could be replicated in other areas nationwide.

Objectives, target audiences and research

The Local Action Group established four key strategies:

1 foster the empowerment of those living with schizophrenia and their family members;
2 include representatives from target groups to help build teams, design strategies for action, and then implement the interventions;
3 work in cooperation with other organizations and institutions to help build a coalition around mental health issues;
4 stimulate volunteer collaboration and collective work.

The Group then developed a series of objectives to address these strategies:

• Develop informational materials and communication programmes.
• Establish the Brazilian Schizophrenia Association (ABRE – Associação Brasileira de familiares, amigos e portadores de Esquizofrenia), the first support group dedicated to those living with schizophrenia, their families and caregivers.
• Promote educational meetings and workshops for those living with schizophrenia, their families and caregivers, as well as mental health professionals and religious leaders.
• Support cultural projects aimed at combating prejudice and discrimination and facilitating social inclusion of persons with schizophrenia, to help foster creativity and communication skills.
• Create a research group and stimulate investigation projects in the field of stigma and schizophrenia.

As part of the first objective, a Communications Strategy Group was created involving mental health professionals, patients and their families, and communication consultants. Together the team created a name for the Brazilian Project (Projeto S.O.eSq) and a logo.

The Local Action Group chose the following target groups for their interventions: patients and family members, journalists and the media, mental health professionals and religious leaders and their communities. Representatives from each of these groups were invited to join members of the Local Action Group in helping to shape and implement interventions. By 2003, S.O.eSq involved 30 active volunteer collaborators.

In 2003, under the direction of Professor Miguel Jorge, a research team from UNIFESP translated and adapted research tools used by other Local Action Groups involved in the global anti-stigma programme, including Canada. The group then began preparing research protocols to cover a number of areas:

• surveys of the general public, health professionals, religious leaders and educators, regarding their knowledge and attitudes;

- content analyses of newspaper and magazine articles on schizophrenia and stigma;
- focus groups with patients and their families on issues of self-stigma and quality of life;
- overall evaluation of the educational activities and communication strategies within the Brazilian Project.

Educational initiatives

Throughout 2002, a team of mental health professionals, individuals living with schizophrenia and family members met and developed content for a series of educational meetings. These included a 12-week educational programme for families and caregivers, which included 15 participants. A larger, open Educational Meeting involved roughly 250 people – those living with schizophrenia, their family members, caregivers and representatives from the clergy.

Partial results from the 222 evaluation forms completed at three educational meetings of these groups showed that:

- 63% reported a significant increase in knowledge;
- 33% reported an increase in knowledge;
- 1% reported no change in knowledge.

In terms of self-reported attitude change:

- 86% reported a more positive attitude;
- 14% reported no attitude change;
- And no one reported a negative change in attitudes.

With the successful establishment of ABRE, the team began implementing educational/support meetings for families and caregivers twice a month starting in March 2003. These meetings and presentations continue to this day.

A Communications Team developed an informational folder and Treatment Resources Directory for patients and relatives, as well as a shorter informational pamphlet that could be used with the general public. The group also developed the S.O.eSq web site, www.soesq.org.br, and a booklet for journalists.

Another on-going informational tool targeted to mental health professionals is the 'S.O.eSq Corner', a regular column in the Brazilian Psychiatric Association Quarterly Bulletin (Psiquiatria Hoje).

Building a coalition

In September 2002, S.O.eSq brought five non-governmental organizations (NGOs) together to meet and discuss the building of a Coalition Movement for Mental

Health in Brazil. The groups began meeting on a monthly basis and continues to build strategies for improving the awareness of mental health issues in both the larger health care community and government. The group was also able to extend its working partnership with UNIFESP to include the Human Resource and Training Center at the State Health Department (CEDRHU).

With financial support from Eli Lilly Brasil and the Brazilian Psychiatric Association, S.O.eSq established an office, staffed by volunteers, in São Paulo.

Cultural activities

In 2001, the Local Action Group initiated the 'Book Project' designed to compile stories from those living with schizophrenia, their families and mental health professionals. Authors described the onset, crisis and diagnosis, treatment and recovery from their own perspective. Targeted to the general public, the book is designed to inform and describe pathways for assistance and support.

In 2002, Dr Cecilia Villares, Rita Narciso Kawamata and Luiz Ribeiro a Brazilian journalist, established the S.O.eSq Writing Workshop to help potential contributors to the Book Project develop their writing skills. The coordinators brought in a variety of different texts, including poems (from authors, such as Carlos Drummond de Andrade, Manoel de Barros and Fernando Pessoa), memoirs (from Fernando Sabino), folklore (Patativa do Assaré) and more informational articles about schizophrenia. Song lyrics, short stories and Japanese haikus were also presented.

Workshops were held between February and November of 2002 with patients and family members. Workshops typically began with distribution of a photocopy of the text. The participants first read the text in silence. Then, the text would be read out loud by all participants. Following that reading, the coordinators posed questions and encouraged open conversation about their interpretations of the text. Insights from this discussion were then applied to the final step during which each participant writing his or her own piece. Some workshops dealt with special topics, such as the movie *A Beautiful Mind*.

In May 2003, members of the workshop extended their exercises to meet, discuss and develop a movie screenplay. These and other workshop participants have spoken of the positive effect the writing exercises have had on reducing self-stigma and giving them a greater feeling of empowerment in their day-to-day life.

Conclusion

The efforts in São Paulo have yet to be fully analyzed though some research has been published. What is clear, however, is that the Local Action Group has:

(a) built upon and extended an existing infrastructure through UNIFESP;

(b) applied the talents and skills of its volunteers in shaping anti-stigma initiatives, such as the Book Project and Writing Workshop.

The ABRE support group has grown in membership to 125 and it continues to establish new partnerships with other family associations and NGOs. Working in partnership with Familiae, a family therapy institute in São Paulo, the groups have developed an 8-week workshop which involves mental health professionals, those living with mental illness and their family members.

For more information on the Partnership Programme in Brazil, please contact

- Cecília Villares (Coordinator)
  UNIFESP
  Departamento de Psiquiatria
  R. Botucatu, 740-3o andar
  São Paulo – SP
  04023-900 Brazil
  Phone/Fax: (+55-11) 5081 3502
  E-mail: cvillares@psiquiatria.epm.br
- Miguel Roberto Jorge (Advisor)
  UNIFESP
  Clinical Psychiatry Section
  Rua Antonio Felicio, 85
  Sao Paulo – SP
  04530-060 Brazil
  Phone: (+55-11) 3079 0262
  Fax: (+55-11) 3079 9232
  E-mail: migueljorge@psiquiatria.epm.br

BIBLIOGRAPHY – BRAZIL

Ludermir, A.B. and Harpham, T. (1998). Urbanization and mental health in Brazil: social and economic dimensions. *Health & Place*, **4**(3), 223–232.

Moreira, M.S., Crippa, J.A. and Zuardi, A.W. (2002). [Social performance expectations in psychiatric patients of a general hospital ward.] [Portuguese] Expectativa de desempenho social de pacientes psiquiatricos internados em hospital geral. *Revista de Saude Publica*, **36**(6), 734–742.

Villares, C.C. and Sartorius, N. (2003). Challenging the stigma of schizophrenia. *Revista Brasileira de Psiquiatria*, **25**(1), 1–2.

14

Egypt

According to the World Health Organization (WHO), in 1999, the population of Egypt was roughly 60,000,000. Of the 120,000 doctors, only 500 (0.4%) of these were psychiatrists (including those in training). Less than one in ten hospital beds in Egypt are reserved for psychiatric patients with roughly one bed for every 7000 Egyptians.

The World Psychiatric Association (WPA) anti-stigma initiative undertaken in Egypt was first organized in Ismailia, located on Lake Timsah, midway between Port Said and Suez, east of Cairo. The Governate consists of five cities – Ismailia, Fayed, Al-Tal, Al-Kabeer, west Qantara and east Qantara. Roughly 700,000 people live in the urban and rural areas of the governate.

One of the first research projects undertaken by the Local Action Group was an assessment of the understanding of the word 'fusam'. Although sometimes the word 'schizophrenia' is written in Arabic, *Al-Fusam* is the term most commonly associated with the illness described in Diagnostic and Statistical Manual for Metal Disorders (DSM) IV and International Classification of Diseases (ICD)-10 as schizophrenia, and is commonly used in textbooks and the mass media.

The first programme coordinator was Dr M. Hassib El-Defrawi working with colleagues in the Neuropsychiatry Department in Ismailia. The group coordinated efforts with the local consumer organization, the local branch of the Rotary Club, and the Association for Health and Environmental Development (AHED).

Research

Much of the early work in Egypt was conducted to assess the knowledge and attitudes of a wide range of groups. Focus groups and small-scale surveys were conducted with: individuals living with schizophrenia and family members, community leaders, primary health care physicians, family physicians, mental health care workers, undergraduate medical students, nurses, psychiatrists, social workers, students and teachers, media personnel, and religious leaders and clergy (both Muslim and Christian).

Primary care physicians

In five rural and urban health care centres in Ismailia, 56 primary care physicians were surveyed regarding their knowledge and attitudes regarding psychiatric medication. While 73% of the general practitioners (GPs) surveyed considered anti-psychotic drugs to be the best method for treating severe mental illness, 64% reported fear that patients might become dependent on these drugs. A full 77% avoid prescribing these medications.

Individuals living with schizophrenia and family members

Two hundred individuals diagnosed with schizophrenia and their families were interviewed. They reported neighbours and the community in general as stigmatizing. Even among family members – while 87.5% expressed support – 62.5% said they would not marry someone with mental illness. Seventy-five per cent of family members believed anti-psychotic medication led to addiction.

A similar proportion (77.5%) reported having made use of traditional treatment methods. For 59%, these non-psychiatric methods were the first attempt at treatment. Among the cultural and traditional interventions reported were: use of the Qur'an (82.7%); herbs and plants (25.8%); Hegab (the practice of writing on pieces of paper; 20.7%) and dietary restrictions (15.5%). Nearly one-third (31%) reported using cautery with hot iron.

Journalists

Focus group discussions with 49 people working in local media found 79.6% would refuse to marry someone with schizophrenia. Seventy-three per cent said they would probably be afraid to speak to them; while 55% said they would not offer them a job.

Interventions

To provide people living with schizophrenia and family members with the latest information on the diagnosis, management and treatment of the illness, a 'Patients and Family Guide' was created. The brochure also addressed relapse prevention. A booklet entitled 'Dignity of Patients with Schizophrenia in the Bible' was created for, and distributed to, Christian clergy. A companion volume, 'Dignity of Patients with Schizophrenia in Islam and Qur'an' was developed for Muslim clergy.

The group also held seminars with key religious leaders and clergy. Members of the media were invited to these seminars which resulted in coverage in the Egyptian print media and on radio and television.

Working with medical students

Another unique aspect of the Local Action Group efforts in Ismailia is its reliance upon the involvement of medical students in anti-stigma research and interventions. These medical students participated in a survey of a group of Bedouins, carried out in 2001. Researchers found that 89% did not recognize the term *Al-Fusam*, used for schizophrenia and 66.6% refused to work with a person known to have a mental disorder.

Students have assisted in developing educational materials, such as videos, brochures, posters and a web site in Arabic. The active involvement of medical students with individuals living with schizophrenia and family members was useful because it:

(a) helped a programme with limited resources that relied upon voluntary contributions;
(b) also reduced fear and stigma of the medical students.

In Ismailia, medical students are encouraged to participate in a 2-week health education project, Schizophrenia Awareness and Reducing Stigma, in local secondary schools. Research still needs to be conducted as to the long-term impact of these efforts.

Secondary school students

In 2000, the Local Action Group in Egypt launched three mental health initiatives to secondary school students in Ismailia and surrounding regions. This educational effort, promoting schizophrenia awareness, reached more than 3000 students, roughly 25% of all those enrolled in grades 10 and 11.

Using research instruments similar to those used in Canada, post-test results showed a remarkable increase in knowledge about schizophrenia from 31% to 84%. Knowledge of treatment options rose from 32% to 69%. In the post-test analysis, students who considered people with schizophrenia dangerous dropped from 81% to 26%.

Broadening the programme

In 2001, under the guidance of Dr Ahmed Okasha, then president-elect of the WPA, the programme was expanded to include the Ministry of Health, Office of Mental Health. Hussein Fahmy, a popular Arab actor, participated with Dr Okasha in a high-profile media event entitled: 'The Role of Mass Media in Elimination of the Stigma of Mental Illness'.

The departure of the director of the Local Action Group in 2001 caused a significant disruption in the anti-stigma efforts. This is one example of why the WPA Global Programme recommends a leadership structure for Local Action Groups that are not solely reliant upon a single individual for internal organization and external relationships (to professionals and organizations).

Through the efforts of Dr Tarek Okasha, the programme continues to broaden its reach.

For more information on the Global Programme in Egypt, please contact

- Tarek Okasha (Coordinator)
  Institute of Psychiatry, Faculty of Medicine, Ain Shams University,
  3, Shawarby Street, Kasr El Nil
  Cairo, Egypt
  Phone: (+20-2) 336 6799/335 0233
  Fax: (+20-2) 748 1786
  E-mail: tokasha@internetegypt.com
- Ahmed Okasha (Advisor)
  Institute of Psychiatry, Ain Shams University
  3, Shawarby Street, Kasr-el-Nil
  Cairo, Egypt
  Phone: (+20-2) 336 6799/335 0605
  Fax: (+20-2) 748 1786
  E-mail: aokasha@internetegypt.com

BIBLIOGRAPHY – EGYPT

El-Shatury, M.H., Ghada, S., Eldin, A.H., Abdelimoneum Maram, M., Radwan, M.A., Elabban Monira, T., Ismail, M.M., Ellabban Nahla, H., Kebeer, A.A., Abdalla and Hassib El-Defrawi, M. (1999). Knowledge and attitude of Bedouins of Saint Catterine towards mental disorders. *The Egyptian Journal of Psychiatry*, **22**(2), 287–294.

Okasha, A. (1995). Settings for learning: the community beyond. *Medical Education*, **29**(Suppl. 1), 112–115.

Okasha, A. (1997). The future of medical education and teaching: a psychiatric perspective. *American Journal of Psychiatry*, **154**(Suppl. 6), 77–85.

Okasha, A. (1999a). Comments on teaching psychiatry to undergraduates. *Israel Journal of Psychiatry & Related Sciences*, **36**(4), 293–296.

Okasha, A. (1999b). Mental health in the Middle East: an Egyptian perspective. *Clinical Psychology Review*, **19**(8), 917–933.

Okasha, A. (1999c). Mental health services in the Arab world. *Eastern Mediterranean Health Journal*, **5**(2), 223–230 [erratum appears in *Eastern Mediterranean Health Journal* 2000, **5**(5), 1059].

Okasha, A. (2001). Egyptian contribution to the concept of mental health. *Eastern Mediterranean Health Journal*, **7**(3), 377–380.

Okasha, A. (2003). Psychiatric research in an international perspective. The role of WPA. *Acta Psychiatrica Scandinavica*, **107**(2), 81–84.

15

Morocco

At the Northwestern corner of the African continent, Morocco, half the size of Egypt ($446{,}500\,\mathrm{km}^2$) is home to roughly 30,000,000 people. Ninety-eight per cent of the population is Muslim. Fifty-three per cent live in urban centres. However, the country has just 300 psychiatrists working in academic, as well as private and public hospitals.

To implement an anti-stigma programme in a country where psychiatric services are so heavily burdened, the World Psychiatric Association (WPA) Advisor, Dr Driss Moussaoui, and Local Action Group Coordinator, Dr Nadia Kadri, enlisted the services of a variety of different professionals, including a member of Parliament, a key representative from the Moroccan Ministry of Health, a psychologist, psychiatric nurses, and representatives from non-governmental organizations (NGOs) such as Chourouq (a family support group for relatives of those living with mental illness) and Nassim (a group dedicated to prevention of substance abuse).

In December 2000, the group established itself as a national programme, called IDMAJ. Both the medical media and pharmaceutical industry have provided support for the initiative in the last 4 years.

Research

As with the work in Egypt, IDMAJ sought to establish a baseline of knowledge and attitudes regarding schizophrenia, and the use of the Arabic term 'Al-Fusam'. Results in Morocco mirror those in Egypt.

Family members and individuals living with schizophrenia

As in other developing countries, research in Morocco has indicated significant involvement of the family in the lives of patients. One hundred individuals with schizophrenia were interviewed at outpatient clinics at the University Psychiatric Center and Berrechid Hospital in Casablanca. Three of four (75%) reported that they had been hospitalized three times or more. A majority reported having lost jobs and friends. Of the 100, 95 reported that they lived with their families throughout the duration of the illness (more than 10 years).

Three of four family members (76%) knew nothing about the diagnosis of 'schizophrenia' or its Arabic counterpart '*Al-Fusam*'. Half (53.1%), however, reported that the illness of their family members was organic or due to brain disease. Many reported that they would not let their family members leave the community or hold a job. Like family members in Egypt, Moroccans reported that neighbours were often the most stigmatizing and difficult to deal with.

Medical professionals

In the survey of 100 general practitioners regarding their knowledge of schizophrenia and attitudes towards those living with the illness 89% reported that they were consulted by mentally ill patients. Two per cent said they refused to consult with patients who were mentally ill. This number rose to 35% when a patient was agitated. One-half required the presence of another person in the room during the consultation.

While a number reported having a family member with schizophrenia (e.g. 11% reported a parent), this had a negative impact on their attitudes towards others with the same illness. Although all reported learning of the illness through their studies, this awareness appeared to provide no protector effect.

Ninety-nine per cent said they would not allow their child to marry a person with schizophrenia (56.2% said that it would cause a 'bad life'). Six per cent reported a fear of having a grandchild with the illness to the shame associated with it.

Interventions

Based on these results, the members of IDMAJ reasoned that information alone would not be sufficient to fight the stigma associated with schizophrenia. One of the first interventions was the creation of weekly meetings with patients in in-patient settings in hospitals to explore the topic of stigma and how best to fight it. The groups explore coping strategies for both patients and family members.

In 2002/2003, focus groups were conducted at the Ibn Rushd University Center in Casablanca to explore the first-hand experiences of stigma and its effects on prognosis of the illness. The focus groups revealed three dimensions of the stigma:

- *The image of the illness itself.* For example, 'aggressiveness' and 'dangerousness' were traits often associated with schizophrenia.

- *The stigma of interpersonal interactions.* For example, the 'social isolation' reported by both those living with the illness and family members.
- *Structural discrimination.* For example, those living with schizophrenia reported lack of rehabilitation systems as being the greatest form of structural discrimination. Family members rated the quality of the available care as of primary concern.

From this data, IDMAJ concluded that it must first educate individuals living with schizophrenia and family members about the illness, about available treatment regimens and about ways to improve the quality of life of those living with schizophrenia. Part of this effort includes social activism. IDMAJ has written to the Chairman of the Moroccan Parliament concerning the availability of medications, the rights of the mentally ill, and their treatment by police and officials in the penal system.

IDMAJ also works in close collaboration with two family associations specifically focused on schizophrenia. Together the groups sponsor a seminar on the stigma associated with schizophrenia.

In December 2001, the 'Lingue Casablancaise pour la santé Mentale', a meeting on mental health in Morocco was held for the twenty-third year. The subject of that year's meeting was 'NO to discrimination against people with schizophrenia'. Five hundred people attended, including: mental health professionals, people living with schizophrenia family members and representatives from associations as well as members of the general public. Many family members spoke publicly for the first time about the suffering caused by the stigma and discrimination because of schizophrenia.

Since that meeting, efforts in Morocco have been expanded to include Marrakesh and Rabat. A 90-min television programme was broadcast on the main network of Moroccan television. The programme included participation of family members who have shared their experiences publicly, as well as more general information on mental health, mental illness and its associated stigma.

In 2002 and 2003, the Local Action Group also conducted a study of written media for the general public. They analysed three daily newspapers – two of them in French (*Le Matin* and *L'Opinion*) and one in Arabic (*Assabah*). They also analysed two weekly newspapers (*Gazette du Maroc* and *Aujourd'hui le Maroc*) and two magazines (*Femme du Maroc* and *Tel Quel*).

Of the 11,600 articles analysed, only 56 (less than half of one per cent, 0.48%) discussed mental illness or mental health, and 14 of these (0.12%) described those with mental illness as being aggressive and unpredictable.

On-going focus on medical professionals

Recognizing the strong stigma that exists in the medical profession, IDMAJ has also developed a series of interventions including a journal article that has appeared in *Esperance Medicale*, a journal for general practitioners. Other journal articles on the work conducted in Morocco have appeared in the international journals *Acta Psychiatrica Scandinavica*, the *Canadian Journal of Psychiatry*, as well as *Social Psychiatry* and *Epidemiological Psychiatry*.

To expand the dissemination of the anti-stigma message beyond the pages of professionals journals, IDMAJ hosts an on-line Forum Discussion at the web site of the Maghrebian *Journal of Psychiatry*. The group has also sought involvement from other associations providing support and services for the mentally ill (e.g. ambulatory mental health care).

Conclusion

Both of the examples from Africa point to the importance of further education to the medical community. At the same time, support networks need to be strengthened for individuals living with schizophrenia and family members, given the current burden on psychiatric services in these countries. Clearly stigma and discrimination are placing pressure on families where the understanding of schizophrenia, its course and treatment is limited.

For more information on the Global Programme in Morocco, please contact

- Nadia Kadri (Coordinator)
  Centre Psychiatrique Universitaire Ibn Rushd
  Rue Tarik Ibn Ziad
  Casablanca, Morocco
  Phone/Fax: (+212-2) 220 6867
  E-mail: n.kadri@casanet.net.ma
- Driss Moussaoui (Advisor)
  Centre Psychiatrique Universitaire Ibn Rushd
  Rue Tarik Ibn Ziad
  Casablanca, Morocco
  Phone: (+212-2) 220 4102/222 8719
  Fax: (+212-2) 296 5125
  E-mail: psych@casanet.net.ma

BIBLIOGRAPHY – MOROCCO

Green, C.A., Fenn, D.S., Moussaoui, D., Kadri, N. and Hoffman, W.F. (2001). Quality of life in treated and never-treated schizophrenic patients. *Acta Psychiatrica Scandinavica*, **103**(2), 131–142.

Moussaoui, D. (2000). What do we gain from collaboration between developing and industrialized countries? *Seishin Shinkeigaku Zasshi – Psychiatria et Neurologia Japonica*, **102**(12), 1209–1216.

16

United Kingdom

As the World Psychiatric Association (WPA) Programme continued to establish new Local Action Groups in new countries in 1998, Professors Graham Thornicroft, Peter Huxley and Vanessa Pinfold of the Institute of Psychiatry were in conversations with the National Schizophrenia Fellowship in the UK (since that time, the National Schizophrenia Fellowship has been renamed Rethink Mental Illness). Dr Pinfold describes the challenges faced with anti-stigma efforts in her country:

In the UK, there are many initiatives to fight stigma and discrimination because of mental illness – both at a national level through government mental health promotion campaigns and voluntary sector groups, and at a local level, using targeted programmes. Very few of these initiatives, however, are ever thoroughly evaluated. The WPA Programme in the UK, based firstly in West Kent sought to develop and evaluate educational anti-stigma interventions with several target groups.

The WPA Global Programme offered a framework to investigate the challenges of fighting stigma and discrimination, while operating in dialogue and comparing results with other members of the global effort. To systematically assess their own effort, the coordinators of the Local Action Group established a three-phase approach.

The first phase, scheduled for August 2000 to January 2002, was to introduce a targeted campaign in West Kent. Based on successful results of that intervention, the programme would be expanded to four other sites in the UK with an evaluation of results in August 2003. Given the results of that phase, the Local Action Group would then seek additional funding to broaden the campaign still further.

A programme Steering Committee was formed and included: politicians, journalists, academicians, individuals living with schizophrenia, family members, mental health promotion experts and representatives of Rethink. They called the initiative: Mental Health Awareness in Action.

Phase One

West Kent is a county in Southeast England. Three target groups were selected from the community of 1,329,652 (2001 census):

- secondary school students averaging 14 years of age;

- police officers;
- other groups including Citizen Advice Bureau volunteers, school nurses and Local Borough Council staff.

The Local Action Group worked in partnership with Maidstone Mental Health Awareness Group, Sevenoaks and Area Mental Health Awareness Group, and the local chapter of Rethink Severe Mental Illness. A systematic training programme was developed and presented to 600 secondary school students and 200 police officers.

Before training was undertaken, however, focus group research was conducted to establish a set of core messages for the systematic training. These core messages were:

- People *do* recover from mental health problems.
- We all have mental health needs.
- One in four people in a lifetime will seek help for a mental health problem.
- Schizophrenia is not a split personality.
- Anyone can be violent – violence is not a symptom of mental illness.
- Mental health problems differ from learning difficulties.

The programmes were evaluated using pre- and post-test survey questionnaires as well as subjective evaluation forms.

Implementing workshops with police officers

Police workshops were designed to provide officers with the skills and confidence necessary to support people with mental health problems who are in distress. Using case studies, participants discussed how to handle particular incidents. Once exercise simulated the experience of 'hearing voices'.

Individuals living with schizophrenia and family members spoke to officers about how the police helped them. They described how the police can be viewed by people with mental illness and what they can do in addition to help people with mental health problems in a variety of situations.

Implementing workshops in schools

The approach taken with students in schools differed from that undertaken with police officers. One of the key goals was to make mental health and mental illness part of the school curriculum, to make it as important in classes as sex and relationships, physical exercise and nutrition, life skills, and drug and alcohol lessons.

These carefully planned educational sessions discussed what mental illnesses are rather than what people suppose them to be. Students are asked to reflect upon the language used to stereotype people with mental illness problems.

Students were given a variety of informational resources and encouraged to seek help from friends or family members, schoolteachers or school nurses, or general practitioners if they are experiencing symptoms. The students also watched an informational video. After the video, consumers answered students' questions often in lively exchanges.

Findings and recommendations

The results of these educational initiatives have been published in the *British Journal of Psychiatry and Social Psychiatry* and *Psychiatric Epidemiology*. More detailed findings of the anti-stigma initiative can be found in these articles. A report entitled 'How Can We Make Mental Health Education Work? Examples of a Successful Local Mental Health Programme Challenging Stigma and Discrimination' is also available. For a copy of the report, contact v.pinfold@iop.kcl.ac.uk

Overall the findings from the initiative in West Kent included:

- Educational workshops can have a small but positive impact on peoples' attitudes towards people with mental health problems.
- Women are more receptive than men to the educational workshops – in both the police and young persons samples.
- Improvements in knowledge about mental illness are weakened over time but the impact of hearing personal experiences are reported to be longer lasting.
- People with personal experiences of mental illness hold more positive views than those without personal experiences – through family, friends or work colleagues.
- Young people who have personal experiences learn more from the workshops than those that report no personal connection with the topic of mental illness.

Based on these findings, the Local Action Group recommended:

- Mental Health Awareness Groups should develop specific aims and objectives, and ensure that all participants are in agreement over the direction and aims of the project.
- Mental Health Awareness Groups should think carefully about the approach they are taking to counter stigma and discrimination, and adopt a framework that reflects their aims and objectives – medical model, disability rights model, recovery model or individual growth model.
- People with mental health problems should be involved in the planning and delivery of mental health awareness workshops – and some programmes will be user-led initiatives.
- The intervention programme should be developed in partnership with stake-holders from the target audience.

- Principles of educational learning theory should be adopted when planning the educational sessions, for example, interactive strategies requiring active learning.
- Long-term sustainability of programmes must be addressed in planning any project.

Phase Two

Having assessed the efforts in West Kent, the Local Action Group then approached Mental Health Awareness Groups in Southern England and extended an offer to implement the educational programmes with their target audiences.

One of the goals of Phase Two was to develop new evaluation tools to assess changes in attitudes, knowledge and behaviour. Another goal was to assess the impact of programmes undertaken by other groups. To date, work has been completed on programmes with the Citizens Advice Bureau, Housing Association and tutors in a London College.

As part of the on-going effort to assess the most effective anti-stigma interventions, the Local Action Group organized a national UK stigma conference on 26 June 2003 in Birmingham, England. The conference was entitled: '*Reducing Psychiatric Stigma and Discrimination: What Works?*' and showcased best practice examples of anti-discrimination projects in mental health. People living with schizophrenia and family members, policy makers, researchers and professionals working in the field of mental health gathered to share examples of current best practice.

Finalization of Phase Two and implementation of Phase Three were scheduled for 2004. As of this writing the group continues to seek funding to carry on its efforts to evaluate the effectiveness of anti-stigma initiatives. Working with Rethink and a consumer-led project based at mental health media, the Local Action Group continues to develop proposals, pursue grants, and work in partnership with other European initiatives to develop tools and methodologies for more effective interventions.

Conclusion

In the UK, anti-discrimination campaigns, such as the one sponsored by the National Institute for Mental Health in England (www.mindout.net) and the Royal College of Psychiatrists (www.changingminds.co.uk) had already been established when the WPA programme began. A national policy framework was already in place, requiring all health and social care agencies to strategically promote mental health for all. This same policy directly calls upon these agencies to combat psychiatric stigma and discrimination across a range of community settings with at risk and vulnerable groups.

Yet prior to efforts by Mental Health Awareness in Action – and other research-based initiatives – assessment results were often unavailable. In some cases, funds may have covered anti-stigma communications but not the research to measure their effectiveness.

In West Kent, the group initiated educational programmes which have provided clear results, and more important, recommendations for moving forward in the future.

For more information on the Partnership Programme in the United Kingdom, please contact

- Vanessa Pinfold (Coordinator)
  Health Services Research Department, Institute of Psychiatry
  P.O. Box 29
  De Crespigny Park, Denmark Hill
  London SE5 8AF, UK
  Phone: (+44-0) 20 7848 0457
  Fax: (+44-0) 7277 1462
  E-mail: v.pinfold@iop.kcl.ac.uk
- Graham Thornicroft (Advisor)
  Head, Health Services Research Department
  Section of Community Psychiatry (PRiSM)
  Institute of Psychiatry at The Maudsley
  De Crespigny Park
  London SE5 8AF, UK
  Phone: (+44-0) 20 7848 0735
  Fax: (+44-0) 7277 1462
  E-mail: g.thornicroft@iop.kcl.ac.uk

BIBLIOGRAPHY – UNITED KINGDOM

Becker, T., Knapp, M., Knudsen, H.C., Schene, A., Tansella, M., Thornicroft, G. and Vazquez-Barquero, J.L. (1999). The EPSILON study of schizophrenia in five European countries. Design and methodology for standardising outcome measures and comparing patterns of care and service costs. *British Journal of Psychiatry*, **175**, 514–521.

Becker, T., Knapp, M., Knudsen, H.C., Schene, A. H., Tansella, M., Thornicroft, G. and Vazquez-Barquero, J.L. (2000). Aims, outcome measures, study sites and patient sample. EPSILON Study European Psychiatric Services: Inputs Linked to Outcome Domains and Needs. *British Journal of Psychiatry, Supplementum*, **39**, s1–s7.

Canvin, K., Bartlett, A. and Pinfold, V. (2002). A 'bittersweet pill to swallow': learning from mental health service users' responses to compulsory community care in England. *Health and Social Care in the Community*, **10**(5), 361–369.

Hatfield, B., Shaw, J., Pinfold, V., Bindman, J., Evans, S., Huxley, P. and Thornicroft, G. (2001). Managing severe mental illness in the community using the Mental Health Act 1983: a comparison of supervised discharge and guardianship in England. *Social Psychiatry and Psychiatric Epidemiology*, **10**, 508–515.

Huxley, P. and Thornicroft, G. (2003). Social inclusion, social quality and mental illness. *British Journal of Psychiatry*, **182**, 289–290.

Leff, J. (2000). Family work for schizophrenia: practical application. *Acta Psychiatrica Scandinavica, Supplementum*, **102**(407), 78–82.

Leff, J. (2002). Science and society: the psychiatric revolution: care in the community. *Nature Reviews Neuroscience*, **3**(10), 821–824.

Pinfold, V. (2000). 'Building up safe havens … around the world': users' experiences of living in the community with mental health problems. *Health and Place*, **6**(3), 201–212.

Pinfold, V. (2002). 'Inclusion in the whole of life: community safety'. In Bates, P. ed. *Working for Inclusion: Making Social Inclusion a Reality for People With Severe Mental Health Problems*, London, Sainsbury Centre for Mental Health.

Pinfold, V. (2003a). Awareness in action: challenging discriminatory and negative attitudes to mental illness should start at school. *Mental Health Care Today*, 24–27.

Pinfold, V. (2003b). How Can We Make Mental Health Education Work? *Example of a Successful Local Mental Health Programme Challenging Stigma and Discrimination*. London, Rethink Publications.

Pinfold, V. (2004). Anti-discrimination actions in mental health. *Journal of Psychiatric and Mental Health Nursing*, **11**(3), 250–252.

Pinfold, V., Bindman, J., Thornicroft, G., Franklin, D. and Hatfield, B. (2001). Persuading the persuadable: evaluating compulsory treatment in England using supervised discharge orders. *Social Psychiatry and Psychiatric Epidemiology*, **36**(5), 260–266.

Pinfold, V., Huxley, P., Thornicroft, G., Farmer, P., Toulmin, H. and Graham, T. (2003a). Reducing psychiatric stigma and discrimination – evaluating an educational intervention with the police force in England. *Social Psychiatry and Psychiatric Epidemiology*, **38**(6), 337–344.

Pinfold, V., Toulmin, H., Thornicroft, G., Huxley, P., Farmer, P. and Graham, T. (2003b). Reducing psychiatric stigma and discrimination: evaluation of educational interventions in UK secondary schools. *British Journal of Psychiatry*, **182**, 342–346.

Ruggeri, M., Lasalvia, A., Bisoffi, G., Thornicroft, G., Vazquez-Barquero, J.L., Becker, T., Knapp, M., Knudsen, H.C., Schene, A., Tansella, M. and EPSILON Study Group. (2003). Satisfaction with mental health services among people with schizophrenia in five European sites: results from the EPSILON Study. *Schizophrenia Bulletin*, **29**(2), 229–245.

van Wijngaarden, B., Schene, A., Koeter, M., Becker, T., Knapp, M., Knudsen, H.C., Tansella, M., Thornicroft, G., Vazquez-Barquero, J.L., Lasalvia, A., Leese, M. and EPSILON Study Group. (2003). People with schizophrenia in five countries: conceptual similarities and intercultural differences in family caregiving. *Schizophrenia Bulletin*, **29**(3), 573–586.

17

Working in Partnership – Australia

The Schizophrenia Australia Foundation was founded in 1986. In 1996, the same year the World Psychiatric Association (WPA) began its global programme to fight the stigma and discrimination because of schizophrenia, the foundation changed its name to SANE Australia. Recognizing the value of sharing information and best practices in their efforts, the WPA global programme and SANE Australia have worked in partnership for nearly a decade, promoting anti-stigma strategies and tactics at seminars and congresses around the world.[1]

Barbara Hocking, Executive Director of SANE, has worked in collaboration with Dr Alan Rosen of the WPA on a variety of initiatives. The goal of SANE Australia is to: 'promote the interest of people with mental illness and educate the general community through the media.' They have established their own information resources for the media, as well as for those living with mental illness, their families and caregivers. They have also achieved significant success in working in collaboration with the media.

A wealth of information resources

SANE Australia published a news magazine, SANE News, which has included articles on issues such as the Social Costs of Mental Illness, Drug and Alcohol Abuse, as well as Art and Mental Illness. These articles are archived on the SANE website: www.sane.org

The website also includes resources such as fact sheets on mental illness, an information portal that lets visitors post questions on mental illness, and press releases on stigma issues in the news. A Charter campaign at the web site also encourages individuals to sign a Charter calling for action to end stigma and discrimination because of mental illness. The Charter has been signed by notable

---

[1] The Mental Health Foundation of New Zealand has also had a successful long-term programme to fight stigma and discrimination. Called 'Like Minds Like Mine', the programme is targeted to all mental illness and is a government-funded campaign managed by the Ministry of Health.

Australians such as the Olympic gold-medallist, Dawn Fraser, international rock star, Peter Garrett, and Archbishop Peter Hollingworth.

The SANE StigmaWatch Programme proactively identifies and addresses stigmatizing depictions of those with mental illness in the news and entertainment industries. Their phone and letter writing campaigns have been successful in stopping the distribution of computer games that referred to the mentally ill as 'a twisted little tribe of freaks' and 'maniacal killers'. In 2000, the group was successful in encouraging the distributors of the movie 'Me, Myself and Irene' to remove stigmatizing language from the packaging of the video release.

SANE is an active member of the Media and Mental Health group set up by the federal government. This group has been responsible for the development and dissemination through media briefings of a press kit entitled: *Reporting Suicide and Mental Illness, a resource for media professionals*. SANE has also produced a video, 'Stigma, Mental Illness and the Media', which includes interviews touching upon the effects of media portrayals on those living with mental illness. The video is another resource used in briefings of journalists and members of the media.

The group's website also has a bookshop that includes recommended books, audio- and videotapes, and CD-ROM educational kits.

In collaboration with the media

Many of the elements described above are designed as correctives for the misinformation disseminated by the media. However, another strategy that SANE Australia has employed has been the active promotion of a realistic portrayal of a character with mental illness in a popular television series. SANE Australia worked with writers of the series on accurately portraying symptoms of the illness and describing various treatment options. The actor and his character were featured on information booklets and pamphlets. The network also provided a link from the programme's website to the SANE Australia website.

Award-winning efforts

In December 2003, SANE Australia received the Human Rights Community Award from Australia's Human Rights and Equal Opportunity Commission for the efforts described above. In September of the same year, the group received the Award for Exceptional Contribution to Mental Health Services at the Mental Health Services Conference in Canberra.

SANE Australia, its Executive Director, Barbara Hocking, and Board Member, Alan Rosen continue to join the WPA in presentations around the world on the fight against the stigma and discrimination because of schizophrenia.

For more information on the Partnership Programme in Australia, please contact

- Barbara Hocking (Coordinator)
  Executive Director, SANE Australia
  P.O. Box 226
  South Melbourne
  Victoria 3124, Australia
  Phone: (+61-3) 9682 5933
  Fax: (+61-3) 9682 5944
  E-mail: barbara.hocking@sane.org
- Alan Rosen
  Mental Health Services
  Royal North Shore Hospital and Community Mental Health Services
  55 Hercules Street
  Chatswood, NSW 2067, Australia
  E-mail: arosen@doh.health.nsw.gov.au

18

Chile, India and Romania

Not every Local Action Group secures the funding it seeks. Not every programme coordinator is able to stay with a programme for 2, 3 or 4 years. People move. Alliances shift. Some programmes may stall as new funding or personnel are secured.

In this chapter we will examine three countries where programmes have yet to achieve the kind of critical mass other programmes have achieved for sustained anti-stigma efforts. One feature stressed over and over by members of the Global Programme Steering Committee is that the Open the Doors programme is not a campaign.

Campaigns tend to be short-term initiatives – limited in scope, time or funding. Unfortunately, the stigma and discrimination because of schizophrenia is not a short-term problem. One very real negative of campaign approaches is that they can raise hopes of the participants in the short term. Consumers and family members, who commit to these effects and see initial interest from politicians or the community at large, may watch as the course of a 'campaign' ends and things return to status quo.

The following examples are of Local Action Groups that have begun initiatives (e.g. executed the first phase of research with focus groups) but have been unable to develop beyond a geographic area, link up to other efforts in other parts of the country, or sustain the initial momentum. All three of these initiatives prepared reports and presentations for the World Psychiatric Association (WPA) World Congress in 2002 but have since undergone significant changes.

Chile

In the late 1970s and 1980s, the dictator Augusto Pinochet dismantled the Chilean National Health Service. During the decades that followed with the introduction of the privatized Isapre health care system, service for low-income families fell precipitously and mental health services overall declined.

With the passing of Pinochet, a number of health care reforms have been under-taken. A report by the World Health Organization (WHO) found that relative to the published national plans for mental health in other countries in Latin America: 'Mexico and Chile are, so far, the best examples of the use of more thorough indicators, and scientific and technical foundations' (Bulletin of WHO 2000, 784).

In 2001, initial efforts focused on two districts in the metropolitan centre of San-tiago, including the San Joaquin district (population: 114,017) and the Santiago district (population: 229,596). A Local Action Group was formed including repre-sentatives from the Health Services of both San Joaquin and Santiago, the University of Santiago, the Association of Families, the Mental Health Unit of the Ministry of Health, and the Chilean Society of Neurology, Psychiatry and Neurosurgery.

One of the first decisions of the group was to undertake surveys of knowledge and attitudes from a wide range of groups: high school teachers, offices of the General Hospital, officials from non-governmental social organizations, police, Ministry of Health officials, medical students at the University of Santiago and family members.

One measure of the public attitudes – or at least of the media's influence on those attitudes – was an analysis conducted by two newspapers in Chile: *Las Últimas Noticias* and *La Nación*. In *Las Últimas Noticias*, a newspaper with a daily circulation of 150,000, 2555 news items were reviewed. Researchers found 157 texts directly or indirectly related to persons that suffer from mental illness.

In *La Nación*, with a daily circulation of 30,000, 2598 articles were reviewed with 99 (3.4%) involving individuals that suffered from mental illness.

Researchers found that in terms of context of the stories these items fell into one of five categories:

- Reports of violence to others.
- Reports of violence to oneself.
- Reports that presented the individual in a 'comic' light.
- Articles offering information on mental illness.
- Reports not related to the mental illness.

Interventions in the psychiatric community

On 12 February 2002, the Chilean Ministry of Health issued Resolution No. 375, a resolution supporting the work of the Local Action Group in reducing stigma due to schizophrenia. That year, four organizations were engaged to assist in interventions in the medical community: Psychiatric Service in the Regional Hospital in Iquique, the School of Nurses of Iquique, the Qualification Programme on Addiction in Puerto Montt and Youth Psychiatry Services at the Hospital 'Barros Luco Trudeau'.

Educational programmes focusing on stigma were presented to psychiatric service teams in the district of Santiago, as well as to the Social Psychiatry Commission of the Society of Neurology, Psychiatry and Neurosurgery. A symposium addressing 'Stigma and Esquizofrenia' was held in Health Region IX.

Educational programmes were also undertaken with social workers involved in serving the Santiago community – both at the General Hospital and in the district itself. Stigma-related presentations were also given to fifth year medical students at the University of Santiago.

Consumers and family members

In 2002, the group also hosted a meeting of family members at the Hospital of Castro to discuss issues surrounding stigma and discrimination because of schizophrenia. The group also hosted a national meeting of family members at La Serena.

With the departure of the key coordinator, the programme has been on hold since 2003. The WPA hopes that new organizers working with the infrastructure of organizations already established in Santiago – and with the support of the Ministry of Health with Resolution No. 375 – can reinvigorate anti-stigma efforts in Chile.

For more information on the Global Programme in Chile, please contact

- Carlos Caceres Gonzalez
  Pampa Engañadora 3168
  Iquique, Chile
  Phone: (+057) 328762
  E-mail: carloscaceres2000@hotmail.com

REFERENCE – CHILE

Bulletin of the World Health Organization (2000). **78**(4).

BIBLIOGRAPHY – CHILE

Alarcón, R.D. and Aguilar-Gaxiola, S.A. (2000). Mental health policy developments in Latin America. *Bulletin of the World Health Organization*, World Health Organization, **78**(4), 483–490.

Navarro, V. (2000). Assessment of the World Health Report 2000. *The Lancet*, 356, 1598–1601.

Vicente, B., Vielma, M., Jenner, F.A., Mezzina, R. and Lliapas, I. (1993a). Attitudes of professional mental health workers to psychiatry. *International Journal of Social Psychiatry*, **39**(2), 131–141.

Vicente, B., Vielma, M., Jenner, F.A., Mezzina, R. and Lliapas, I. (1993b). Users' satisfaction with mental health services. *International Journal of Social Psychiatry*, **39**(2), 121–130.

Santigotimes, Public Health Care system in the spotlight study reveals performance often does not meet international standards, 8 May 2001, CHIP News.

The Times of India, Wealth of Ill-Health, 24 June, 2000, Bennett, Coleman & Co Ltd.

Santiago Times, Over a Third of Chileans Suffer from Mental Illness, 3 July, 2001, CHIP News.

India

While a few of the programmes in this volume have been ambitious enough to start as national initiatives as opposed to expanding outward from a single metropolitan area, the challenge of initiating a national programme in the second most populous country on the planet begs for a word beyond 'daunting'.

The country is divided into 28 states – each with its own health care delivery service. The population in India now tops 1 billion – served by fewer than 4000 psychiatrists (and many of these in private practice). Today there is roughly one mental health worker (psychiatrist, clinical psychologist or nurse) for every 250,000 people.

In terms of government support of mental health, a report in the *Psychiatric Bulletin* in 2002 notes: 'Although there is a Mental Health Act, use of mental health legislation is virtually non-existent' (Das *et al.*, 2002). Development of community services furthermore 'appear to be low on the priority list of the government and funding is a major issue'.

The importance of family support

Professor Narendra N. Wig, member of the WPA Steering Committee from India, has observed the difference between psychiatry in India and Western countries is the involvement of the family in treatment regimen. 'My colleagues in the West were discussing how successful they were at seeing family members and educating them about schizophrenia.' 'Success' was measured as actively involving 20–25% of the families in treatment of a family member.

'When asked about my experience in India, I find the question of "percentage" to be almost irrelevant. The vast majority of our patients arrive with a family member. These relatives also stay in the wards with patients – assisting us with a number of duties in the care of that person.'

Although this may be changing somewhat with on-going industrialization (Sethia and Chaturvedi, 1992), the involvement of family members is a key feature of Indian psychiatry and an essential component in the study of the stigma associated with schizophrenia.

The National Institute of Mental Health and Neuroscience (NIMHANS) in Bangalore, with the guidance of Dr R. Srinivasa Murthy, sought to coordinate efforts in four major centres in India: Bangalore, Chennai, Delhi and Mumbai. Key to development of the Local Action Groups in each city was the involvement of consumer and family support organizations.

In Chennai, for example, SCARF is a voluntary organization that has been working with consumers living with schizophrenia and their families for more than 15 years. Another group, AASHA, is a family support organization that has developed a self-help approach with city officials.

RAHAT, a volunteer organization involved with issues concerning mental illness and drug dependency, provided support to the local action group in Delhi.

PRERANA is a voluntary support organization in Mumbai involved in suicide prevention. Working with MAITHRI, an initiative that was begun by psychiatrists, the Local Action Group has begun to develop more family support structures within the Mumbai community.

Funding limitations, however, have precluded any epidemiological data from being gathered and compared among the centres. This is not to say that efforts in India were unsuccessful.

From 25–26 May 2001, family members and caregivers from two dozen centres across India participated at a conference in Chennai. The object of this meeting was to provide support and networking so that consumers and family members move from recipients of services to active participants, from being the object of stigma to active, organized opponents.

These family organizations have begun to work with international service organizations such as the Rotary and Lions Clubs to develop further employment opportunities for consumers. These family groups now run special awareness programmes on stigma during events such as World Health Day, Mental Health Week and World Disabled Day. Family groups have also become more active in public rallies, seeking improved services for individuals with physical and mental disabilities.

New initiatives

On 6 February 2004, Dr Abdul Kalam, President of India, helped launch a renewed anti-stigma effort in India – that includes a collaboration between SCARF and the WPA Global Programme. The President spoke to university students gathered at the Music Academy in Chennai. At the event, he asked students to take an oath not to stigmatize or discriminate against the mentally ill.

The event was covered by both the print and broadcast media. Since then, a short film has been developed in Tamil and English for educating students in high schools and universities.

In recognition of World Schizophrenia Day on 24 May 2004, SCARF organized a number of other activities for the public:

- Articles on schizophrenia were published in newspapers that included: *The Hindu, Anna Nagar Times* and *Dina Mani.*

- A message about schizophrenia was printed on milk packets sold in markets for the general public.
- Pamphlets about World Schizophrenia Day and schizophrenia were distributed at hospitals and shopping malls.
- A programme of interviews of psychiatrists and those living with schizophrenia was broadcast on Podhigai television in prime time. The participants discussed the first-hand experience of the stigma and discrimination because of schizophrenia.

World Schizophrenia Day also marked the start of a new support programme called SHAPES (Society of Hope, Action, Empathy and Regard for Schizophrenia), started by patients and family members.

Educational initiatives

Awareness programmes on mental health and mental illness have been conducted in 10 schools and colleges in Chennai. Working with Sowmanasya Hospital, educational programmes were held in 13 other colleges (including the Colleges of Nursing, Social Work and Engineering). To date, 4000 students have participated in these programmes.

Working with the National Service Scheme

The National Service Scheme (NSS) organizes awareness programmes in schools and colleges on a broad range of social issues and enlists support for volunteer activities in the community. Working in cooperation with members of the NSS, the Chennai Local Action Group has been able to 'train the trainers' to disseminate more information to the general public on mental illness. NSS leagues in colleges adopt villages in neighbouring districts and conduct volunteer social service activities. The goal is to create an educational network built upon mutual trust and community service.

This networking with social groups will continue with educational programmes to law enforcement personnel, as well as social support organizations in rural communities around Chennai including Kattangulathur, Minjur and Karlapakkam. Perhaps one of the most important educational initiatives planned, given the importance of the family doctor in early detection and diagnosis of mental illness, is for medical students and general practitioners.

With successful implementation in and around Chennai, SCARF plans on working with other major urban and rural communities in a broader network to combat the stigma and discrimination because of schizophrenia.

For more information on the Global Programme in India, please contact

- R. Thara
  Schizophrenia Research Foundation
  R/7A, North Main Road
  West Anna Nagar Extension
  Chennai 600 101, Tamil Nadu, India
  Tel: (+91-044) 26153971, 26151073
  E-mail: scarf @ vsnl.com

BIBLIOGRAPHY – INDIA

Das, M., Gupta, N. and Dutta, K. (2002). Psychiatric training in India. *Psychiatric Bulletin*, 26, 70–72.

Harrison, G., Hopper, K., Craig, T., Laska, E., Siegel, C., Wanderling, J., Dube, K.C., Ganev, K., Giel, R., an der Heiden, W., Holmberg, S.K., Janca, A., Lee, P.W., Leon, C.A., Malhotra, S., Marsella, A.J., Nakane, Y., Sartorius, N., Shen, Y., Skoda, C., Thara, R., Tsirkin, S.J., Varma, V.K., Walsh, D. and Wiersma, D. (2001). Recovery from psychotic illness: a 15- and 25-year international follow-up study. *British Journal of Psychiatry*, 178, 506–517.

James, S., Chisholm, D., Murthy, R.S., Kumar, K.K., Sekar, K., Saeed, K. and Mubbashar, M. (2002). Demand for, access to and use of community mental health care: lessons from a demonstration project in India and Pakistan. *International Journal of Social Psychiatry*, 48(3), 163–176.

Mojtabai, R., Varma, V.K., Malhotra, S., Mattoo, S.K., Misra, A.K., Wig, N.N. and Susser, E. (2001). Mortality and long-term course in schizophrenia with a poor 2-year course: a study in a developing country. *British Journal of Psychiatry*, 178(1), 71–75.

Murthy, R.S. (1998). Rural psychiatry in developing countries. *Psychiatric Services*, 49(7), 967–969.

Murthy, R.S. (2000). Community resources for mental health care in India. Epidemiologia *e Psichiatria Sociale*, 9(2), 89–92.

Murthy, R.S. and Burns, B.J. (eds) (1992). *Proceedings of the Indo-US Symposium on Community Mental Health*, Sponsored by National Institute of Mental Health and Neuro Sciences, Bangalore: NIMHANS.

Samuel, M. and Thyloth, M. (2002). Caregivers' roles in India. *Psychiatric Services*, 53(3), 346–347.

Schulze, H. (1999). Schizophrenia stigma and discrimination: an India perspective. *OpenDoors, The Newsletter for the Global Schizophrenia Awareness Program*, Vol. 2.

Sethi, B.B. and Chaturvedi, P.K. (1992). Family and social support systems in the case of the mentally ill. In: Murthy, R.S. and Burns, B.J., eds. *Proceedings of the Indo-US Symposium on Community Mental Health*. Sponsored by National Institute of Mental Health, Neuro Sciences. Bangalore: NIMHANS, pp. 277–288.

Srinivasan, T.N. and Thara, R. (1997). How do men with schizophrenia fare at work? A follow-up study from India. *Schizophrenia Research*, **25**(2), 149–154.

Srinivasan, T.N. and Thara, R. (1999). The long-term home-making functioning of women with schizophrenia. *Schizophrenia Research*, **35**(1), 97–98.

Srinivasan, T.N. and Thara, R. (2001). Beliefs about causation of schizophrenia: do Indian families believe in supernatural causes? *Social Psychiatry and Psychiatric Epidemiology*, **36**(3), 134–140.

Thara, R., Kamath, S. and Kumar, S. (2003a). Women with schizophrenia and broken marriages – doubly disadvantaged? Part I: patient perspective. *International Journal of Social Psychiatry*, **49**(3), 225–232.

Thara, R., Kamath, S. and Kumar, S. (2003b). Women with schizophrenia and broken marriages – doubly disadvantaged? Part II: family perspective. *International Journal of Social Psychiatry*, **49**(3), 233–240.

Thara, R., Padmavati, R. and Srinivasan, T.N. (2004). Focus on psychiatry in India. *British Journal of Psychiatry*, 184, 366–373.

Thara, R. and Srinivasan, T.N. (1997). Outcome of marriage in schizophrenia. *Social Psychiatry and Psychiatric Epidemiology*, **32**(7), 416–420.

Thara, R. and Srinivasan, T.N. (2000). How stigmatising is schizophrenia in India? *International Journal of Social Psychiatry*, **46**(2), 135–141.

Romania

The WHO Report on Mental Health in Europe (2001) reported that 'in the last 5–6 years there has been an increasing acceptance for both patients' rights and psychiatric ethics (in Romania)'. However, the 'list of shortcomings which need to be addressed' was formidable:

- Lack of up-to-date comprehensive studies on morbidity or studies evaluating population needs within a definite area or with certain risk factors.
- Lack of (or only a rudimentary level of) multidisciplinary teams for out-patients, due to the reduced number (or even absence) of persons and/or necessary positions (psychologists, social workers, vocational therapists and legal advisors).
- The development of social protection and non-medical ways of helping some categories of mentally ill patients and some populations with a high risk for mental illness.
- Insufficient day centres and counselling services (of various types).
- Lack of effective coordination of the care services at the national level.
- Postgraduate specialist training is still based on an excessively biological and reductionism model, which seems to promote pharmacotherapy as the only really effective and credible therapeutic approach. Continuing education is inadequate.

- Liaison psychiatry, forensic psychiatry, community psychiatry and psychotherapy are not officially recognized.
- The general practitioners and other specialists lack basic psychiatric knowledge and have little capacity to provide psychiatric help or make referrals to psychiatrists.

In October 2001, a national anti-stigma programme was announced. The Local Action Group consisted of psychiatrists and mental health care workers and included the president of the Romanian League for Mental Health. The programme received official recognition from the Romanian Academy, the Minister of Health, and the Prime Minister. Eli Lilly – Romania provided logistical and financial support.

For the country of roughly 22.5 million, the Local Action Group defined five long-term programme objectives:

- To evaluate existing mental health policy.
- To increase positive media presentations on issues concerning schizophrenia.
- To maintain and update the national database of the League for Mental Health.
- To increase the number of professionals involved in the Local Action Groups.
- To organize regular conferences on schizophrenia, and the stigma and discrimination that accompany it.

In 2002, a number of interventions were undertaken including workshops with students in secondary schools, active involvement with journalists and the media to disseminate anti-stigma messages, and exhibitions of the poetry and artwork of those living with mental illness. Six centres in five cities throughout Romania began working with theatre groups to develop productions that would dramatize issues of stigma and discrimination due to mental illness.

For reasons unknown to the WPA Programme Steering Committee, little information is available as to why the initiatives yielded no data beyond the interventions cited above. While certain key coordinators appear to have moved on from the programme it is unclear if the national ambitions of the effort outstripped available financial resources or the time of volunteers involved.

For more information on the Global Programme in Romania, please contact

- Raluca Nica (Coordinator)
  Romanian League for Mental Health
  Sos. Mihai Bravu 90-96, Bl D17, Sc 4, Ap 149 Sector 2
  Bucharest, Romania
  Phone/Fax: (+40-1) 252 0866
  E-mail: lrsm@dnt.ro

- Bogdna Tudorache (Advisor)
  President, Romanian League for Mental Health
  Sos. Mihai Bravu 90-96, B1 D17, Sc 4, Ap 149 Sector 2
  Bucharest, Romania
  Phone/Fax: (+40-1) 252 0866

REFERENCES – ROMANIA

WHO (1996). *Health Care Systems in Transition: Romania.* Copenhagen: World Health Organization Regional Office for Europe.

WHO (2001). *Mental Health in Europe.* Country reports from the WHO European Network on Mental Health.

19

Conclusions and Recommendations

One of the key, and compared to many other anti-stigma efforts, unique elements to the success of the local action initiatives described in this volume is collaboration: that is, collaboration among those living with schizophrenia, their families and support groups, medical professionals, government officials and other experts. From the first-person perspective of the patient or family member to the expertise of a public relations professional, each Local Action Group brings together a variety of perspectives.

As an *international* initiative, the anti-stigma programme of the World Psychiatric Association (WPA) has been able to offer its participants four advantages.

First, Local Action Groups in 20 countries have developed *nearly 200 interventions* to a wide range of target groups. As we will see in comparisons later in this chapter, results from these interventions can be compared and contrasted to determine new, more effective ways forward.

Second, the WPA Programme has allowed each new group that joins to learn from earlier efforts following the same methodology. For example, members of the Partnership Programme from Calgary, Canada have met with groups in Europe and Latin America to develop strategies for educating and changing attitudes of children in secondary schools. Similarly, the family support group, Schizophrenia Research Foundation (SCARF), in Chennai has been able to share its experiences with other nascent family support groups in other countries. In addition to these exchanges, there were two International Conferences focused on the Stigma and Discrimination because of Schizophrenia – the first held in Leipzig, Germany and the second held in Kingston, Canada – have served as instructional forums and networking opportunities for the diffusion of best practices.

Third, *intra*-country cooperation has also benefited from the WPA international alliances. By joining the WPA global effort, Local Action Groups have been able to extend their own reach and involvement and, in essence, to broaden the table for participating groups in a country. Governmental and non-governmental organizations that had not worked together found common ground in this international programme. In West Kent (UK) and Calgary (Canada), family support organizations that had worked separately in the same city (in one case, across the street from each other) came together and worked side-by-side for the first time.

Fourth, all of the material prepared by the global programme – from the step-by-step guide in Volume I to the stigma bibliography – have served as central resources. The experience gained and tools used in earlier interventions were applied to later efforts. In their work with medical professionals in Spain, the Local Action Group there published Volume II as a stand-alone reference book on schizophrenia, its treatment and issues surrounding stigma and discrimination.

The global web site, *www.openthedoors.com*, has been translated from English into Arabic, German, Greek, Italian, Japanese, Portugese and Spanish. This web site provides an overview of the objectives and participants in the programme. More important, it also contains information from Volume II of the programme materials described above. For those living with the illness and their families, the web site also contains educational material taken from a training manual developed by the Local Action Group in Calgary, Canada. Visitors to the web site are also able to download electronic versions of the programme volumes as well as informational brochures developed for different target groups. A password-protected Intranet site was also made available for programme participants to share information in a less public forum than the Internet.

Statistical analysis of web site traffic from 1999 to 2001 found that visitors from different countries increased dramatically – sometimes 100-fold – when a Local Action Group was established in that country. Factoring out the disproportionate traffic from the US during the first few years of the programme, the greatest number of visitors were from Canada, Spain and Germany, where Local Action Groups were in place.

Structure and flexibility

Volume I of the programme materials specified a very particular methodology for development of the Local Action Group and implementation. Yet these guide-lines were flexible enough to allow each site to act upon local opportunities and address any local limitations. In the final analysis, the work of these centres was as operationally similar as the countries were culturally different.

One example is how initiatives moved from local to national in scope. The majority of programmes sought to first establish a local presence in one city or metropolitan region (e.g. Madrid) or several (e.g. Sendai, Tokachi and Okayama) before taking the programme nationally.

Some programmes, by design or limitation of resources, did not diffuse beyond their initial target communities (e.g. Boulder, Colorado in the US). Yet, even these programmes had elements that extended beyond any set geographical boundary.

In Boulder, for example, the training course for law enforcement officials and judges is being used in other communities in the US.

Since those guidelines were first developed, the WPA Anti-stigma Programme has also developed a training manual to help countries interested in starting their own programme. This training manual has been distributed at workshops at scientific conferences and contains more specific information on such topics as: 'How to conduct focus group research' and 'Selection of target audiences'.

Overall, the model of successfully implementing a local initiative before extending that work nationally is the approach recommended by the authors of this volume. *How* one diffuses the programme nationally is a function of resources and time. Initiatives of this programme that have a national reach are generally of three types.

Both Poland and Greece began with strong organizing groups in a major metropolitan area – Krakow and Athens, respectively. While few anti-stigma efforts will have the advantage of having one of its chief organizers appointed Minister of Health, as in the case of Greece, what both of these nationally successful groups share is a central organizing committee with more than one individual responsible for key decisions.

The national anti-stigma effort in Germany benefited from the fact that one of the chief organizers, Professor Wolfgang Gaebel, was also a member of the National Schizophrenia Research Network. His office in Düsseldorf was the central reporting centre for seven other sites in this network, each site developing its own unique intervention. The collective results from the nationwide initiative have yet to be compiled and published, but preliminary results from some of Professor Gaebel's work and others are available. (See references for Chapter 5 on Germany.)

Austria and Romania are examples of a third type of national effort which relied upon a central organizing group to implement a single, coordinated national initiative from the very outset. In the case of Austria, the national effort was implemented through the development and distribution of mass media messages, followed by more targeted interventions in select high schools. Romania took a national approach, distributing its messages in pamphlet and booklet form, through the established national network of a family support organization.

When and how to move from local intervention to national initiative will vary from country to country and rely upon available structures, such as the reach of national support organizations or governmental assistance. However, five things appear to be necessary to make a successful transition:

1 An established model, tested on a local level which can be implemented in other communities (e.g. education of psychiatrists in Spain).
2 A central organizing group to whom regional teams report on a regular basis.

3 Some continuity of leadership, involving one or more of the original participants from the successful local initiative in the larger national effort.

4 Clear, on-going communication between these regional groups and the central organizing group, and conversely, a sense of involvement by the regional groups and vision of the national goals of their efforts.

5 A long-term commitment to the programme as a *programme*, not as a short-term campaign; too often, campaigns raise expectations of those who have dedicated their time and may leave those with long-term interests in on-going success (e.g. patients or family members) disappointed when funding or momentum are exhausted.

As in the case of Germany, Poland and Spain, the plan to expand the programme nationally was present in initial planning stages of the Local Action Group. While most groups may begin with aspirations for regional, national or international success, it will be important to build the framework for that success even as the local foundations are being laid.

Target groups

Table 19.1 is a compilation of target groups identified by various Local Action Groups of the WPA Programme. General practitioners and other health care professionals were chosen by every country save Poland, US and UK. As the first point of medical consultation for both patients and their families, they have been clearly identified as being one of the groups most in need of anti-stigma interventions (with psychiatrists and mental health professionals not far behind).

A close second was the target group of journalists and the media. These choices are notable both because the target groups are sources of information to others (e.g. family members or the general public) and because how they speak about the illness and the individual can have an impact on self-stigma as well. (For more evidence of the importance of these target groups to those living with schizophrenia and their families, see the Focus Group.)

Another target group identified by 13 of the 18 sites listed in Table 19.1 was secondary school students. Reasons cited for this choice include the fact that first episodes of the illness may appear in the late teens and that this group can be reached through educational programmes in schools. Other reasons for selecting this group were the inverse relationship between age and attitudes regarding mental illness (older adults showed greater social distance and were more difficult to reach as a group) and the fact that younger individuals often become enthusiastic supports of work against stigma (e.g. as students demonstrated in Egypt).

Table 19.1 Target audiences

	Consumers	Family members and friends	Primary and/or secondary education	Medical students	Psychiatrists and mental health professionals	General practitioners and other health care professionals	Journalists and the media	General public	Government workers and non-governmental agencies	Religious communities and clergy	Businesses and employers	Judicial and law enforcement officials, lawyers
Austria		✓	✓		✓	✓	✓	✓				
Brazil	✓	✓			✓	✓	✓	✓	✓	✓		
Canada	✓	✓	✓	✓	✓	✓	✓	✓	✓	✓	✓	
Chile					✓	✓	✓	✓				
Egypt		✓	✓	✓		✓	✓			✓		
Germany	✓	✓	✓		✓	✓	✓	✓			✓	
Greece	✓	✓	✓		✓	✓	✓	✓		✓		
India	✓	✓	✓			✓	✓					
Italy	✓	✓	✓		✓	✓	✓	✓		✓	✓	
Japan	✓	✓	✓		✓	✓			✓			
Morocco	✓	✓	✓		✓	✓	✓	✓				
Poland	✓	✓	✓		✓	✓	✓	✓	✓	✓	✓	
Romania	✓	✓	✓		✓	✓	✓	✓				
Slovakia	✓	✓	✓		✓	✓	✓	✓				
Spain	✓	✓	✓		✓	✓	✓	✓				
Turkey	✓	✓	✓	✓	✓	✓	✓	✓				
UK		✓	✓			✓	✓		✓			✓
US	✓	✓	✓			✓	✓	✓			✓	✓

Due to the global nature of this programme, when early evidence from the Partnership Programme in Canada showed marked improvement in knowledge and attitudes with this target group, other groups used the model and adapted the methodologies to their own cultural realities. Fay Herrick from the Partnership Programme in Calgary has served as a consultant with other centres over the years.

As explained in Chapter 4, the Local Action Group in Spain developed the 'inside-out model' for implementation, working with the immediate circle of influencers on the patient and his or her family. For that reason, the group chose psychiatric professionals as one of their initial target groups. The goal would be to extend efforts outward over time as stigma is reduced and as resources allow.

This concentric model showing families and psychiatrists as closest to the patient influence and gradually radiating out to more distant influencers (and potential stigmatizers) may explain several relationships between the choice of target groups and socioeconomic data. That is, the nine countries with the lowest Gross Domestic Product and fewest psychiatrists per capita chose families as targets for anti-stigma interventions and support.

Conversely, four of the seven countries with the highest Gross Domestic Product per capita targeted businesses and employers. In the case of Boulder, Colorado, working with the local Chamber of Commerce, the Local Action Group had access to the 10 companies employing 90% of the community's workers.

Success of work with any of these selected target groups is dependent upon three factors:

1 The assessment of the first-hand experience of those living with schizophrenia and their family members – or any other group, including medical professionals who may be the objects of stigma and discrimination. Looked at from the point of view of expertise, these individuals and their experiences can provide powerful insights into how stigma is manifested and how it may be addressed. The Focus Group section below outlines findings from seven countries where focus groups were used to assess qualitative information.

2 The involvement of at least one member of the target group in the intervention. By involving members of the target group, these initiatives were able to gain access to other members of the target group as well as develop more effective message and media strategies.

3 The more defined the target audience, the more directly the message and media strategies will address that audience. While most groups identified the 'General public' as one of their targets, placement of messages in any mass medium immediately implies some form of segmentation. For example, radio formats (e.g. talk shows or hip-hop music) and television programmes (e.g. soap operas

or the evening news) skew to certain demographics. The better defined the target audience – for example, 18- to 24-year olds with a high school education – the more effective your message and media choices will be.

Focus groups: results from seven countries

Among the countries participating in the programme at present, seven conducted qualitative studies on the needs and perceptions of people with schizophrenia and family members. In the local needs assessment for WPA Programme activities, focus groups were used in Brazil, Germany, Italy, Morocco, Switzerland, Turkey and UK.

These groups applied the focus group method to achieve five different ends:

- To understand the stigma experiences of people with schizophrenia and their families (Brazil, Germany, Italy, Morocco, Turkey, Switzerland and UK).
- To define and test key messages of the programme (Germany and UK).
- To define relevant target groups (Brazil, Germany and UK).
- Monitoring and on-going process evaluation (Germany, Morocco and Turkey).
- Understanding families' needs for support in crisis situations or at admission to hospital (Morocco).

Considering the substantial variation in cultural context, language, mental health care systems and family structures across the seven programme sites, the general ways in which stigma is affecting the everyday lives of people with schizophrenia and their families are strikingly similar. Differences between the different countries only show at the level of very concrete experiences in a particular field of stigmatization.

Significant similarities also existed between the experiences of stigma and discrimination as reported both by those living with the illness and their family members. For example, both groups identified the social isolation they experienced and the withdrawal of friends and neighbours.

Both groups, in all seven countries, identified negative images in the media, specifically the association of violence with schizophrenia, as being part of their experience of stigma. They also identified lack of information among the general public and public health professionals. Those living with the illness expressed frustration at exclusion from the labour market, while family members spoke to the financial burden resulting from that lack of employment. Family members also reported that they were assigned blame and responsibility for the illness.

The four dimensions of stigma

Overall the focus groups revealed a pattern of four general areas in which stigma is encountered: interpersonal interaction, structural discrimination, public images of mental illness and access to social roles. These dimensions have been revealed in the German focus group study on stigma perception of people with schizophrenia (Schulze and Angermeyer, in press), but appear to be reproduced across the globe.

The first dimension, interpersonal interaction, refers to stigma and discrimination experienced in the context of social relationships. The reduction of social contacts ensuing from problems in the interaction with others is perceived as the central area in which the stigma of schizophrenia is experienced – by service users and families alike.

However, this dimension is the only one based on interpersonal stigma. The three remaining dimensions represent more structural barriers. The stigma of schizophrenia also expresses itself in the situation that the illness represents a major obstacle denying access to important social roles, predominantly in the fields of employment and partnership. Beyond the domain of social interaction, stigma is further experienced through structural imbalances built into legal regulations, health insurance statutes and political decisions, as well as through the stereotypical, largely negative attitudes of the public and the media portrayals reflecting and reinforcing these stereotypes.

While there is agreement between people with schizophrenia, families and mental health professionals about the general dimensions in which stigma is experienced, they vary significantly in the weight they attached to the different dimensions.

Mental health professionals placed public images of mental illness as the single most significant dimension of stigma. However, patients and family members identified interpersonal interactions as the most significant dimension of stigma. Those living with schizophrenia themselves identified access to social roles also as far more significant than either mental health professionals or family members. For family members structural discrimination was a far more important dimension than for either patients or mental health professionals.

Also, aspects of the experiences assume a different meaning, depending upon who describes them and upon the context chosen for recounting an experience. Focus group results show that, with their different foci of attention, patients, relatives and mental health professionals each put emphasis on particular aspects of the problem and view stigmatization in the light of their own everyday experiences and specific interests. This variation supports the WPA approach of considering the perspectives of all groups involved in struggling with schizophrenia in order to get a comprehensive picture of how the stigma attached to the illness affects the patients' quality of life, self-esteem and chances to benefit from optimal treatment services. This more holistic approach allows Local Action Groups to consider aspects of stigma that might not be seen by either group alone.

What should be done? Suggestions for anti-stigma interventions

Stigma experiences of services users and families form the basis for programme development in the WPA effort against stigma. Suggestions for anti-stigma interventions reflect the areas where service users and relatives detected stigma. Four main areas for activities against stigma were identified. A summary of the suggested areas for anti-stigma interventions is given in Figure 19.1.

1 **Public relations – working with the media**
   – Articles in popular newspapers/magazines
   – Festivals, events, workshops, seminars
   – Public relations by psychiatric service institutions
   – Internet, new media
2 **Changes in mental health care**
   – More communication with patients and relatives
   – More out-patient and preventive services
   – More community-based services, better networking
   – Involve users and families in evaluating mental health services
3 **Support for users and families**
   – Training programmes: stigma-coping, empowerment, social competencies
   – More information about schizophrenia/treatment options in lay terms
   – Creation of job opportunities
4 **Education and training**
   – Mental health as a topic in school (for students and teachers)
   – Improvement of psychiatric training
   – Better education about schizophrenia for health professionals, especially general practitioners
   – Training seminars for employers
   – Training seminars for the police and legal professionals

Figure 19.1 What should be done? – Four areas of intervention

Communication messages: Who we are and how we'd like to be seen

Focus groups have also been used to develop and test communication messages for various programme activities. Looking at the way in which people with schizophrenia and their families would like to see themselves portrayed in the WPA Programme, three key messages become apparent from the many suggestions made in the focus groups:

We are people just like you!
Schizophrenia can be treated, and we can live with it!
Stigma hurts. Stigma destroys life chances. Stop it now!

These themes imply the desire to highlight commonalties between those with schizophrenia and the general public, to focus on family roles, hobbies, music preferences, favourite dishes or special sporting successes rather than only on the illness in their public portrayal, and to create an awareness that schizophrenia can affect anyone – something many of those living with the illness would not have believed themselves before the onset of the illness. The focus of the messages also indicates that hope and a perspective for improvement or stability are of great importance in coping with schizophrenia and its consequences, and that achieving a kind of normality seems desirable – both in the patients' own lives and for the image of schizophrenia they would like to see advanced.

Monitoring and process documentation: How do people with schizophrenia benefit?

In Turkey and Germany, focus groups were conducted at regular intervals to assess how service users perceive programme process. For this, the same people who had participated in the focus group session for the needs assessment were invited several times so that they could offer their input as the project developed. A second series of focus groups was carried out with people with schizophrenia who actively participated in various anti-stigma projects to get their views whether and how they actually benefited from their involvement. Identifying needs for support was a second aim of these groups.

While the data is from a very small sample, the initial feedback from participants is encouraging. With increasing duration of their work for the programme, those living with the illness reported a growing self-esteem and confidence, which helped them to challenge stigmatizing behaviour and reject devaluating statements about themselves.

Finally, people with schizophrenia on the project teams learn a lot through their involvement. Many of them even feel that they acquired skills that better qualify them for a job on the first labour market, that they are doing a kind of a traineeship for 'the real world'.

Focus group successes

Focus groups have been a useful tool for the WPA Programme in identifying areas of intervention that reflect the needs and perceptions of those who are exposed to the stigma and know best what stigma means in practical terms. The method with its non-directive approach stimulates communication among group participants rather than predominantly between the facilitator and individual group members. It has also helped to encourage people with schizophrenia and their families to articulate grievances and negative experiences which may otherwise have remained hidden from the views of programme developers due to social desirability.

In addition to understanding the demands on an effective anti-stigma effort, focus groups have also helped to involve service users and families from the start of the programme. The participation of all relevant partners is crucial for programme sustainability and the credibility of communication messages. In addition, some focus group participants stayed with the project and have joined the local action committees and project teams.

Finally, as it appears from the first feedback of service users and family members actively supporting the project, basing an important part of the needs assessment on the perceptions of people with schizophrenia and their carers has helped to ensure that those at the receiving end of stigma benefit from the programme, continue to support it and have developed a sense of ownership which is so important in sustaining a continuous programme to fight stigma and discrimination.

Report prepared by Beate Schulze

A question of media

Table 19.2 presents a list of *almost 200 interventions* undertaken in the various countries participating in the WPA effort. Nearly half of these were educational programmes targeted to children and adolescents, psychiatrists, general practitioners and other health care professionals, journalists, clergy and family members. Research from these initiatives supports earlier findings that targeted community educational efforts are most effective at changing knowledge and attitudes (Wolff *et al.*, 1996).

Nearly every Local Action Group was also able to generate press coverage in newspapers and magazines, both local and national. Editors of these publications are often looking for news stories. Similarly, many reporters are interested in having experts they can contact for news stories that involve mental health issues. Finding these editors and journalists can prove invaluable in future presentations of stories in the news as well as with the effectiveness of stigma watch or stigma-busting efforts.

Table 19.2 Global Activity Report 2003

	Austria	Brazil	Canada	Chile	Germany	Greece	Japan	Italy	Morocco	Poland	Slovakia	Spain	Turkey	UK	US
Survey of knowledge/attitudes	✓	✓	✓		✓	✓	✓	✓	✓	✓	✓	✓	✓	✓	✓
Speaker's bureau	✓	✓	✓		✓		✓	✓		✓	✓	✓	✓	✓	✓
Primary and/or secondary education	✓		✓		✓	✓	✓	✓			✓		✓	✓	
Educating psychiatrists	✓	✓	✓	✓	✓		✓			✓		✓	✓		
Educating GPs	✓		✓	✓	✓							✓	✓		
Educating other health care professionals	✓	✓	✓	✓	✓	✓	✓	✓	✓	✓		✓	✓	✓	
Educating journalists	✓	✓	✓		✓	✓	✓	✓		✓		✓			✓
Stigma Busting/Stigma Watch				✓	✓	✓		✓				✓			✓
Educating clergy		✓	✓			✓		✓		✓					
Publications in scientific journals	✓	✓	✓		✓	✓	✓	✓	✓	✓	✓	✓	✓	✓	✓
Publications in newspapers/magazines	✓	✓	✓		✓	✓	✓	✓	✓	✓	✓	✓	✓	✓	✓

(continued)

Table 19.2 (*continued*)

	Austria	Brazil	Canada	Chile	Germany	Greece	Japan	Italy	Morocco	Poland	Slovakia	Spain	Turkey	UK	US
Radio programmes	✓	✓	✓			✓			✓	✓	✓	✓	✓		✓
Television programmes	✓	✓	✓			✓			✓	✓	✓	✓	✓		✓
Anti-stigma awards	✓	✓			✓	✓						✓			
Theatre/dramaturgic presentations	✓		✓		✓	✓									
Story workshops		✓	✓								✓				
Art presentations/competitions		✓	✓		✓	✓				✓				✓	✓
Educating families	✓	✓	✓			✓			✓	✓	✓	✓		✓	
Other	Education with public Movie screening/festival				Open-Door-Day in the hospital (every year) Benefit: Jazz concert	Benefit: Nana Mouskouri		Focus groups with patients and family members	Educating patients	Day of solidarity with people suffering from schizophrenia	Media cell	Web Site Educating patients Public lectures Media guide	Short films for TV		Books Cinema slides Bus Ads Public lectures

Roughly half of the countries also developed some form of public, cultural event. These included plays, poetry readings and dramaturgical workshops, the joint film project between the German and Slovak groups, as well as high school art competitions in Canada and the US. Brazil, Germany, Greece, and Poland had events corresponding to the release of the movie, *A Beautiful Mind*, specifically.

In Calgary, research indicated that nearly one-third of the respondents to the post-intervention survey recalled having heard radio messages played on local radio stations. In terms of reach of the message, roughly 300,000 people recalled hearing these anti-stigma messages. Dr Ruth Dickson, one of the coordinators of the programme, whose voice was featured in the commercial, reports that a year after the messages were broadcast, patients and family members she met for the first time would comment that they had heard the messages and remembered her name.

However, research conducted soon after the broadcast saw no measurable change positively or negatively in *attitudes*. Some reasons for this might include the negative media coverage of two significant news stories running at the same time (i.e. a subway incident in Toronto and the trial of the Unabomber in the US).

In the case of mass media, two questions remain: while messages such as those created for television in Austria have won awards from the broadcast industry, do messages in the mass media help change public attitudes and improve the lives of those living with schizophrenia?

The second question is a bit more complicated and has to do with the *cumulative* impact of multiple interventions in the community. How might messages work *across* media? Put a different way, how can messages within a community or country work together and achieve certain synergies?

For example, in Boulder, Colorado, to supplement the educational programmes conducted in high schools, the Local Action Group also conducted art competitions with students and featured winning entries on buses students took to and from school. In the summer months, anti-stigma messages were featured in cinemas on slides shown before the feature films.

Consumer advertising research has demonstrated a 'multiplier effect' – where message effectiveness increases when multiple media is used (Smith, 2002). While there is less research on this for social marketing efforts (in part because of the comparatively small amount of money spent on social marketing compared to consumer), it is reasonable to assume the multiplier operates for this form of marketing communications as well.

As the earlier, anecdotal story of Dr Dickson showed and as reports from participants in Local Action Groups indicate (e.g. participants in the film project in Germany and Slovakia), the development of supporting mass media programmes can be both memorable and foster a greater sense of empowerment among those living with the illness and their families.

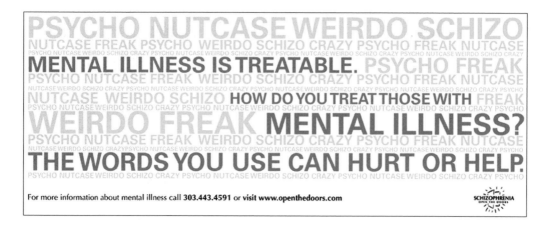

Can we allow targeted educational efforts to tell the whole story? How effective can these efforts ultimately be if a teenager or law enforcement official then leaves the presentation only to receive contrary messages in the media and hears stigmatizing comments from their peers? Certainly, the groundwork made by many of these Local Action Groups to foster deeper relationships with journalists and the media will help ensure continuity of the anti-stigma message. The work being done by media watchdog groups and 'stigma busters' has also put pressure on the owners of print and broadcast media to be attentive to the content of their publications and programming.

Development of messages

Focus groups (described in the sidebar above) helped some of the Local Action Groups identify key messages to communicate. Other groups also used qualitative research to examine knowledge and attitudes of their target audiences in order to identify what myths, misconceptions and discriminatory ideas their audience harboured.

Communication professionals working in the field of consumer marketing know that it is not enough to simply state a fact or competitive benefit of a product or service. They need to answer two other questions: 'Why should I care?' and the call to action, 'What do you want me to do?' These questions are just as important to social marketing.

The figure above shows one of the cinema slides used in Boulder, Colorado during the summer of 2001 as part of the anti-stigma intervention targeted to teenagers. The primary message is that 'Mental illness is treatable'. But this is followed up with a simple question: 'Why should I care?', and the answer is: 'The words you use can help or hurt someone with mental illness', accompanied a series of common, derogatory words for those living with mental illness.

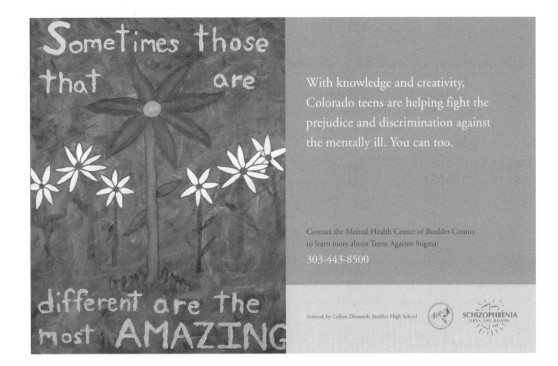

The message to teenagers presented these commonly used words for what they were: derogatory, insults and epithets that constitute a form of discrimination to those with mental illness. The message was crafted in such a way to present the viewer with a choice to assist or continue hurting those with mental illness. The cinema slides also featured a call to action, contact information of where the teenagers might find more information on mental illness.

The following year, winners from the art competition poster contest were displayed on public transportation that students took to and from school, often these were schools where presentations had been conducted on the stigma associated with mental illness. The artwork and messages were prepared by teenagers for their peers.

Research in countries such as Spain raised concerns that brief 30- or 60-s messages might raise more questions and concerns about schizophrenia than they answered. Of all of the factors involved in development of anti-stigma interventions, the development of messages has some of the greatest variability. Not only between countries considering cultural differences, but between target groups *within a single country* where the differences in knowledge and attitudes may be pronounced.

As the programme continues in other countries, the library of anti-stigma materials will continue to grow. A few elements such as the programme logo described below have had a resonance that has translated from one language to another.

A Global Identity

The WPA Global Programme to Fight the Stigma and Discrimination because of Schizophrenia, while being an accurate and descriptive title of the initiative undertaken in 1996, is also a bit unwieldy. Following the first meeting in Geneva, Switzerland, the graphics designer, Mark Jones, working with the authors of this book developed a series of logotypes to work with several different, shorter names.

The Steering Committee of the programme reviewed the names and logotypes and selected, *Open the Doors*, and the logos shown below for several reasons.

The door is a universally recognized symbol for access and admission. There are many different types of doors: to employment, to hospitals, to the homes of both families and friends. The experience of stigma and discrimination for those living with the illness and their families is in some way that of doors once open, now closed.

The active verb 'Open' can be read as request or even command to give access to someone who previously has been shut out.

The brevity of the statement made it more easily translatable than other, longer phrases.

The name and logo were successful beyond expectations. The logo has been translated into 12 languages. It serves as a simple mnemonic for the global web site: *www.openthedoors.com*. It has helped countries with limited resources to use a theme and graphical element to easily identify the programme and the communication materials in a professional manner and through repeated use built greater recognition.

It has been featured on T-shirts and commemorative stamps in Greece. In Poland and Turkey, it has been used as a rallying image for Open the Door Days. In the case of Poland, a large door, set in the main square of Krakow, has served as a gateway through which supporters pass to sign a petition of solidarity for those living with schizophrenia and their families.

In a century when so much information (and some would add: disinformation) is disseminated through so many media, a simple memorable phrase and image can help develop greater recognition and quickly identify disparate communication materials as part of one, unified global effort.

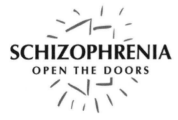

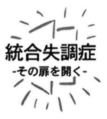

Recommendations about principles of programme development

Over the years, learning from experience and research done in this programme and elsewhere, the WPA has formulated the following principles which are also recommendations to those starting new programmes.

First, the programme has to be long lasting and not a campaign. Profoundly imbedded attitudes and social arrangements including laws cannot be expected to change overnight. Short-lasting paroxysms of public education often leave people who expected a great deal from a campaign more unhappy and dissatisfied after it than before it. Long-lasting special programmes usually become impossible to fund after a while. An anti-stigma programme not only needs to last over time, but also has to devote some its energies to becoming a routine part of health and social service plans and institutions.

Second, a programme against stigma must be successful if it is to retain the loyalty of those who work on it. That means that the goals of the programme have to be stated in broad, overarching terms but that specific plans for immediate application have to be modest in size and ambition. That also means that the goals of the programme must have local relevance.

Third, the programme must deal with the problems experienced by the people who have the illness and their family. While the process of stigmatization is similar in different settings, what bothers people is different. The only way to identify what is the most bothersome – and should therefore be among the goals of the programme – is to ask those who are most directly affected about their experience and about targets that they would see as being most important in terms of improving their situation.

In most parts of the world, there are *not* systematic studies that document consumers' everyday problems and experiences: yet without such data, it is likely that much energy will be spent in action that will give more satisfaction to those who have undertaken it than those whom it was supposed to serve.

Asking consumers and their families about their problems before starting a programme gives the programme the support of those who have been stigmatized. It gives them an opportunity to become actively engaged in efforts that directly affect them.

Fourth, the programme should not be an affair of the mental health service system alone. The participation of others – representatives of different sectors of government and of community members – is not only important because it leads to programme strength. A broad involvement allows interventions in different walks of life by those involved.

In addition, it brings people who are not directly concerned with mental illness in contact with mental health service personnel, with consumers, with their families and with others who are concerned with mental illness. The narrowing of the gap that exist between psychiatry and the rest of medicine and society is of great importance for the survival of the programme and for an improvement of mental health care.

Fifth, the programme should employ those who have had the experience of schizophrenia and their families in day-to-day functions of the programme. As examples from the participating sites show, the active involvement of people who have the experience of having the illness can reveal areas of need that medical professionals might not otherwise have given the greatest priority. Just as important, their active involvement in the programme acts against the loss of self-esteem, a loss that represents a great obstacle and increases self-stigma in any effort to rehabilitate a person who suffered from a mental illness.

Sixth, it has been critical to develop a model that can be easily understood and used both in planning and evaluation of the programme. The vicious circle model that was developed for the WPA Programme is presented above. Its advantage is that it can be used to counteract the reluctance of those involved in supporting a programme against stigma because its main message is that there are numerous entry points. Potential partners in fighting stigma can be shown concrete areas where their expertise can apply in breaking the vicious cycle and different stages of development.

Seventh, one of the many enemies of long-term projects is the fatigue and burnout that leaders of the programme experience. Every effort should therefore be made to add a component to the programme to prevent burnout.

An alternate and additional antidote employed by the WPA Programme has been the involvement of a large number of centres in the programme. Variations in output and energy available to move the programme along, differ among centres and within a single centre. By having multiple centres, it becomes possible to have some of them active and leading at a time when other sites are going through a fallow period.

The fact that the WPA Programme had 20+ centres also contributed energy to the programme by offering possibilities for small-scale collaboration among groups that would otherwise have had difficulty in identifying partners among professional groups (e.g. organizations of patients and their relatives).

Eighth, in addition to using modern technology and linking sites electronically via a web site, the WPA also invested in organizing face-to-face encounters among participants in the programme. Heads of a site that had already completed work served as consultants for new sites. They were invited to report on their experiences at scientific meetings and at annual meetings of participating sites. Newsletters and annual reports were used to record and publicize the work done and to give recognition to achievements of the participants. Exhibits were developed for scientific meetings where the progress of programmes could be placed on display.

Ninth, and finally, a programme has to have tools to help newcomers to the programme and to facilitate the decision of those who might be hesitant in participating. Among the materials produced to aid Local Action Groups in their initiative:

- A volume giving guidelines and a detailed description of the different stages that should be followed and milestones that should be met.
- A description of the work done in different sites of the programme.
- A bibliography of articles and books dealing with stigma focusing on work over the past two decades.
- A listing of papers produced by the programme sites.
- A volume summarizing knowledge about schizophrenia and indicating issues that are of particular importance in preventing or diminishing stigmatization.
- An inventory of posters, videos and other materials used in different countries.
- A manual for programme implementation.
- Standard curricula and syllabi for courses on how to start a programme.

Finally, the most important recommendation that can be made on the grounds of experience from this 10-year effort is that a successful programme against stigmatization and its consequences can be launched in any country – small or large, rich or poor, industrialized or developing – and the success of this work is richly rewarding for all those involved because it gives them the certainty that they have done something that must be done in a civic society. Furthermore, it gives people who suffer from mental illness and those who care for them a new lease on life and hope for a better tomorrow.

REFERENCES

Smith, A. (2002). *Take a Fresh Look at Print*, 2nd edn. International Federation of the Periodical Press (FIPP) and Alan Smith.

Wolff, G., Pathare, S., Craig, T. and Leff, J. (1996). Community attitudes to mental illness. *British Journal of Psychiatry*, **168**(2), 183–190.

Afterword

Living in an age as thoroughly drenched in mass media as we are, it is easy to believe that communicating a message and changing public opinion is simply a matter of resolve. Or money. 'Anyone can compose an advertisement.' 'I've got a bit of a creative streak.' 'How hard can it be to come up with a catchy phrase or rhyme people will remember?'

Mass media itself is largely to blame for this misconception. With so many simple-minded messages that lodge in our minds like stones in our shoes, we might imagine that a clever turn of phrase or dramatic image is all that it takes to capture the attention of a massively distracted (and, in the case of mental illness, massively indifferent) culture. But changing stigma and discrimination because of schizophrenia demands more attention. It requires changing opinions and attitudes. As survey after survey has shown, in country after country, communities are made *aware* of the need for assisted housing or job programmes for those living with mental illness – yet the attitude remains: 'Not in my neighbourhood, not in my company'.

In the nearly 10 years I have worked on the WPA Global Programme against Stigma and Discrimination because of Schizophrenia, three things have become starkly evident to me: the enormity of the challenge facing those living with schizophrenia, and their families and caregivers; the strength and resolve of all of these individuals; and finally, the power of human testimony.

Working and talking with many of the Local Action Groups described in this book, I have been struck (though not surprised) at how, early in the planning stage, conversations turn to using expensive television and radio advertising. But sitting in a classroom watching a young man who has recovered from schizophrenia and a father who has lost a son to suicide, as they speak to rapt teenagers, I have seen how powerful and effective testimonials are. Just as remarkable is the courage these individuals show in relating their often heartbreaking experiences. Listening to the students' questions – sometimes direct and sometimes personal – and responses that elicit a laugh or an awed silence, one can see how human communication *does* change attitudes and behaviour.

The collective and international effort of so many people has made this pro-gramme unique. Journalists, government officials, police officers, medical students, an international opera diva and others worked together with those living with schizophrenia and their families. Through that collaboration and communication, significant changes are taking place. Families have found support where none existed before. Judges have changed sentencing guidelines. High school students are telling their parents about the conversation they had in school with someone who had struggled with mental illness. Small support groups have suddenly found themselves linked to a global network working towards the same goal: to eradicate the stigma and discrimination because of schizophrenia.

Hugh Schulze
Chicago, US 2005

Appendix I
Volume I: Guidelines for programme implementation

Implementation

This part of the programme document describes how to develop and implement a local programme as part of the international effort undertaken by the World Psychiatric Association (WPA) to combat stigma and discrimination because of schizophrenia.

The following chart lists all the steps involved in developing, implementing and evaluating a local programme along with a proposed timetable for completion. Steps that have to be undertaken simultaneously are listed together at the same point on the timetable.

It is anticipated that the implementation of the programme, as indicated in the timetable, will take approximately 2 to 2½ years. It is, of course, recognized that the actual time needed to complete each step may vary from site to site; however, it is recommended that local groups complete each step in the order specified. The timetable is divided into the following major phases:

    I. Preliminary steps
   II. Collection of information about programme site
  III. Designing the programme
  IV. Adaptation, development, pre-testing and revision of programme tools
   V. Implementation and monitoring of the programme
  VI. Evaluation of the programme
 VII. Planning action after programme ends

Weeks	Step	Check box	Date completed
	I. PRELIMINARY STEPS		
0–6	1. Site Selection	❏	_____
7–10	2. Identification of Local Project Coordinator	❏	_____
11–12	3. Briefing of Local Project Coordinator	❏	_____
13–20	4. Establishment of Initial Planning Group	❏	_____
21	5. Planning Group Meets with WPA Representative	❏	_____
22–24	6. Production of First Draft of Local Action Plan	❏	_____
25–28	7. Nomination of Local Action Team Members	❏	_____
29–32	8. Invitation to Local Action Team	❏	_____
33–34	9. First Meeting(s) of Local Action Team	❏	_____
35–38	10. Review of Draft Action Plan	❏	_____
	II. COLLECTION OF INFORMATION ABOUT PROGRAMME SITE		
39–46	11. Development of Site Description	❏	_____
	12. Assessment of National Health/Mental Health Policies and Services	❏	_____
	13. Review of Institutional Capabilities (including currently available mental health services)	❏	_____
	14. Analysis and Description of Communication Resources	❏	_____
	15. Review of Prior and Existing Stigma-Reduction Programmes and Materials	❏	_____
	III. DESIGNING THE PROGRAMME		
47–48	16. Formulation of Long-Term Goals	❏	_____
49–52	17. Formulation of Short-Term, Site-Specific Objectives	❏	_____
	18. Obtain Communication Consultant	❏	_____
	19. Selection of Target Audiences	❏	_____
53–56	20. Agreement on Potential Messages	❏	_____
	21. Selection of Media	❏	_____
57–60	22. Preparation of Work Schedule for Overall Programme and Team Members	❏	_____
	23. Development of an Organizational Chart	❏	_____
	24. Preparation of Budget	❏	_____
	25. Official Recognition from WPA	❏	_____

Weeks	Step	Check box	Date completed
	IV. ADAPTATION, DEVELOPMENT, PRE-TESTING AND REVISION OF PROGRAMME TOOLS		
60–64	26. Baseline Survey	❑	_____
	27. Selection of Available Media Materials	❑	_____
	28. Agreement on Central Theme and Programme Concepts	❑	_____
65–68	29. Development of Message Concepts	❑	_____
	30. Decision on Production of New Materials	❑	_____
69–70	31. Pre-test of Message Concepts	❑	_____
71–78	32. Development of Media Materials	❑	_____
79–80	33. Pre-test of Materials	❑	_____
81–84	34. Finalization of Communication Materials	❑	_____
	V. IMPLEMENTATION AND MONITORING OF THE PROGRAMME		
85–104	35. Building Local Support and Consensus Building	❑	_____
	36. Implementation of Programme by Local Action Team Members	❑	_____
	37. Coordination of Implementation Schedules with All Team Members	❑	_____
	38. Maintenance of Programme Diary	❑	_____
	39. Monitoring	❑	_____
	VI. EVALUATION OF THE PROGRAMME		
105–120	40. Post-Test of Knowledge, Attitudes and Behaviour	❑	_____
	41. Evaluation of Programme	❑	_____
121–129	42. Review of Overall Outcomes	❑	_____
	VII. PLANNING ACTION AFTER PROGRAMME ENDS		
130	43. Assuring Continuation of Work After the End of the Programme	❑	_____
131–134	44. Documenting the Project	❑	_____
	45. Replanning for Future Development (applying the lessons)	❑	_____

I. Preliminary steps

There are two options for using the instructions outlined in this document. In some cases, local groups, psychiatric societies or institutions may want to tailor this programme to their own needs and use it without officially participating in the WPA Programme. We request that groups wishing to use the programme in this way inform the WPA about their efforts and provide appropriate acknowledgement of the WPA materials while conducting their project. Groups interested in becoming an official participating site in the WPA Programme should contact Professor Norman Sartorius at the Département de Psychiatrie, 16–18, Bd de St Georges, 1205 Genève, Switzerland. Being recognized as an official participating site requires an undertaking that:

(a) the programme steps outlined in this document will be followed;
(b) the results of the programme and the experience gained will be fully shared with WPA Member Societies and with other participating sites;
(c) the published materials created as part of this programme should be submitted to the WPA to become a part of the archives of this worldwide programme;
(d) whenever possible, the Local Group should consult with WPA about publications destined for very wide distribution. When more than one programme is operating in a country, consultation between such programmes concerning publications is obligatory;
(e) the use of the WPA programme materials and all help received from the WPA, from donors and other participating sites will be fully acknowledged in all presentations of the programme.

1. Site selection

The following factors should be considered in selecting a site for the programme:

- *Geography*: A working group's efforts should be able to cover the area/region under consideration. Other questions to consider: Do local media cover this specific region? Are there times when the geographical or climatic conditions divide the area or disrupt communication? Are media from other regions likely to disrupt the programme?
- *Language*: Can materials be cost-effectively developed in a single language? Will programme participants be able to communicate using the same language? Are there significant minority group influences? Is the area socially cohesive?
- *Political and economic situation*: Is the site politically unified? Is the central governmental ready to support the programme? How willing are local political and financial entities to initiate and sustain the programme? Are there significant economic variations between different parts of the area?

- *Long-range potential*: Does this effort have a chance to continue in the area and to radiate to other sections of the country? Factors to consider in evaluating this question include: similarity of language; acceptability of results (cultural relevance); the existence of traditional exchanges between the programme area and other areas of the country or other countries.
- *Availability of support*: Are a sufficient number of individuals likely to remain interested in the programme over a long period? Are there institutions or organizations likely to support the programme?

2. Identification of Local Project Coordinator

Once a site has been selected, a local coordinator for the project should be identified who has:

- local acceptability;
- good standing in the community;
- access to an institutional base with a pre-existing infrastructure (e.g. adequate administrative support).

This individual must be willing to commit considerable time and effort to the programme for at least 3 years. It is also helpful if the coordinator or the institution involved has some experience in organizing community programmes.

3. Briefing of Local Project Coordinator

The local coordinator should be briefed about the efforts of the WPA Programme to date. The coordinator should be given materials related to the project and should meet with members of the WPA Resource Group. The local coordinator should also be given the opportunity to visit a site in which the programme is underway. If the group will be officially participating in the WPA Programme, it is the responsibility of the local coordinator to maintain liaison with WPA.

4. Establishment of Initial Planning Group

The local coordinator will convene the Initial Planning Group, which should include a small number of individuals selected on the basis of their interest in the programme and knowledge of the issues involved, and their access to financial and political resources, consumer groups, and relevant local treatment organizations. This group should consist of four to five people (i.e. a number who are able to meet over dinner or travel in the same vehicle). Ability and willingness to work in a team is a key quality, given the long-term nature of the programme.

As soon as the Initial Planning Group is established, the Local Project Coordinator will brief the group on the WPA effort in detail. The briefing should be given to the group when they are gathered together and sufficient time should be allowed to arrive at a common understanding of the project.

5. Planning Group Meets with WPA Representative

After the Initial Planning Group has been briefed on the experience of the project in other countries, key issues important to success and integration with global efforts, a meeting with members of the WPA International Resource Group (IRG) should be organized. The WPA/IRG Representatives should plan on spending approximately 1 week's time with the Initial Planning Group (over a 2- to 3-month period) to ensure continuity and iterative dialogue. It is expected that each new site will have access to two experts of the WPA/IRG.

6. Production of First Draft of Local Action Plan

After this meeting with the WPA/IRG Representatives, the Initial Planning Group should agree on broad objectives and develop a two- to five-page outline of tentative goals and proposed interventions including financial, budgetary and administrative considerations. This document should contain a brief discussion of plans for establishing a Local Action Team. This planning document will then be reviewed by the WPA and future Local Action Team members.

7. Nomination of Local Action Team members

The following groups should be among those considered in selecting possible nominees for the Local Action Team:

- patient and family advocacy groups;
- legal professionals;
- journalists;
- health care professionals;
- legislators;
- influential members of the community (e.g. business leaders, religious leaders, etc.).

In order to best capture full community consensus, the planning group should consider sending invitations to those who might initially be considered adversarial, but whose ultimate involvement will be helpful.

The group should appoint a member of the group to create a programme diary in which the step-by-step process of the group is recorded.

8. Invitation to Local Action Team

Invitations to join the Local Action Team should involve a two-part process:

- a letter of invitation from the Local Project Coordinator;

- a letter from the representative of the WPA Task Force welcoming the member when the invitation is accepted.

The Local Action Team should also begin to develop a wider network of advisors and consultants whom they can call on.

9. First Meeting(s) of Local Action Team

More than one meeting may be required in order to ensure the consensus and commitment of all members to the programme and to develop a single, unified effort. The agenda for the first meeting of the Local Action Team should include:

- opening remarks,
- introduction of participants,
- description of overall WPA stigma-reduction programme and of experiences from other sites engaged in the programme,
- presentation of broad action plan,
- agreement on how the Local Action Group will work,
- tentative timetable of project.

10. Review of Draft Action Plan

The Local Action Team should scrutinize the first draft of the local action plan that was developed by the Initial Planning Group. Enough time should be allowed to discuss and agree on the meaning of the terms used, the implications of the objectives, and the most acceptable ways of intervening in the community. The Team should also try to identify the time required and expected outcome for each step, and create a checklist or worksheet to track their progress. Once this draft action plan has been agreed upon, the group should collect information necessary to adapt the plan to the local situation.

II. Collection of information about programme site

11. Development of Site Description

What follows are broad guidelines for collecting information. This process should involve well-informed members of the community as well as all other available sources of data. It will often be necessary to accept estimates since collecting the data in a systematic manner would be too time consuming. Exactly what information should be collected will depend on its relevance to the project. Note that the demographic information should not be averaged, but should be identified relative to population distribution (e.g. a country's literacy rate averages may hide important difference between urban and rural settings). It may be necessary to augment some of the information gathered with mini-surveys, focus group discussions and other methods of qualitative research. (See Volume I, Appendix A for a sample of the types of information that might be collected.)

After the information is collected, a narrative should be developed. This narrative should be an engaging profile and not simply a list of facts and estimates. It should include reasons for the programme as well as pointers for action (e.g. for selecting target audiences).

The site description should include:

- demographics,
- education,
- economic features,
- geography,
- social characteristics,
- cultural characteristics,
- attitudes toward people with schizophrenia.

12. Assessment of National Health/Mental Health Policies and Services

The team should assess the general health and mental health policies in the site area as well as the health care services that are currently available to those with schizophrenia, including the quality of inpatient facilities. The findings of this survey may be useful in developing messages that target inequalities in the existing health care delivery system. A sample survey of baseline information to be gathered concerning health policies and services is provided in Volume I, Appendix B.

13. Review of Institutional Capabilities (including currently available mental health services)

During the implementation of the programme, it may be possible to involve existing institutions. When this is undertaken, it will be important to establish who is able and willing to speak to target audiences (e.g., an educational authority might speak to teachers; the director of a hospital might speak to the doctors or gather them together for instruction).

14. Analysis and Description of Communication Resources

The purpose of this step is to gather information about available media and communication resources. A list of specific resources to consider is provided in Appendix C to Volume I. This group should examine these resources and determine the most effective way to reach various target groups in the site area (i.e. which media should be used). It is especially helpful to identify and try to make contact with individuals who can be helpful to the project and who may have an interest in it (e.g. media executives and directors; medical editors and commentators for newspapers, and local radio and television stations).

15. Review of Prior and Existing Stigma-Reduction Programmes and Materials

The Local Action Team should amass a full complement of materials suitable for an intervention against stigma that are already in existence in various media (e.g. films, posters, instructional leaflets). These materials should be sought from sources such as community agencies, churches, the health care system, the media, non-government organizations (NGOs), and libraries. A list of materials produced in various countries is available upon request from Professor Norman Sartorius at the Département de Psychiatrie, 16–18, Bd de St Georges, 1205 Genève, Switzerland. The Local Action Team should discuss these objectives and be sure that they have arrived at a common understanding of their meaning, and that they have found them relevant and acceptable for their community.

III. Designing the programme

16. Formulation of Long-Term Goals

After the analysis is completed, the next step is to establish long-term goals relative to awareness, knowledge and action. The overall objectives of the International Programme are:

- to reduce or eliminate stigma and discrimination because of schizophrenia;
- to improve the social acceptance, community integration and quality of life of people with schizophrenia and their families and caregivers;
- to increase the contribution of those with schizophrenia to society.

17. Formulation of Short-Term, Site-Specific Objectives

Short-term, measurable objectives that are specific to the site and relevant to target audiences should be formulated next. These objectives, which will form the basis for assessment of the project, should be specific, realistic, prioritized, and progress towards them should be measurable. They should be formulated in a manner that will allow for an evaluation of the programme and a comparison with baseline (see Step 26).

Each step in designing the programme should be seen as part of an iterative process in which short-term, measurable objectives relate to long-term goals and to specific audiences, messages and media (see Figure A1).

18. Obtain Communication Consultant

It is helpful at this stage to consult someone with communication expertise who has experience in performing surveys and planning media campaigns that are acceptable and successful in this particular community. This individual or company can help the team project the costs of the project (see Step 24).

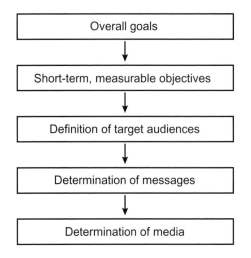

Figure A1.   Sequence of decisions

19. Selection of Target Audiences

The target audiences should be segmented by demographic, geographical, social, psychological or other relevant characteristics as defined in Step 11. Examples of possible target groups include:

- clinical officers/medical assistants;
- community leaders;
- emergency room physicians;
- employers;
- families of people suffering from schizophrenia;
- general physicians;
- landlords;
- medical students and residents;
- nurses;
- police and corrections officers;
- politicians and legislators;
- portions of the general public segmented by age, income or social class;
- psychiatrists;
- social service workers;
- students and teachers;
- traditional healers.

20. Agreement on Potential Messages

The Local Action Team should develop a list of possible messages to be delivered to the target audiences. Messages that overlap relative to the target audiences should be clearly identified. In the process of identifying messages, the group should explore the following:

- Frequent causes of stigma or discrimination (in the setting in which the programme will take place). Some examples of the kinds of stigma and discrimination that occur because of schizophrenia are given in Volume I, Appendix E.
- Reasons for not getting treatment or other help.
- Common myths and misunderstandings.

Four categories of messages should be considered:

- Messages to provide accurate information (e.g. schizophrenia is treatable).
- Messages targeted at an attitude, not a fact; these messages will have a more emotional component (e.g. acceptance of people with schizophrenic illness).
- Messages to improve people's skills in handling situations in which they may encounter people with schizophrenia (e.g. situations in which they would currently be unable to cope with unusual behaviour such as acute excitement in a public place).
- Messages intended to change behaviour (e.g. providing increased access to emergency care or employing a person who has had schizophrenia).

21. Selection of Media

The group should review target audiences to determine which are the most appropriate media to communicate to them. The communication consultant (see Step 18) should be helpful in doing this. Messages should then be reviewed relative to the medium being considered. For example, certain messages might not be appropriate for billboards. The team should do a pilot assessment of the effectiveness of various media for different target audiences (see Volume I, Appendix F).

22. Preparation of Work Schedule for Overall Programme and Team Members

The work schedule should be organized to include the timing and sequence of each proposed action and a schedule for each Local Action Team member. The work plan should also be structured to allow flexibility in implementation. The schedule should include personnel, materials, production schedules, fieldwork training, equipment, travel and evaluation.

The Local Project Coordinator and Action Team should consider ways to ensure that their initial enthusiasm and motivation are maintained. For example, they should identify feedback mechanisms, set up regular meetings and give members full responsibility for specific tasks so that they can feel true ownership of tasks they consider important. Using members of the Action Team as consultants for programmes at other sites may also help maintain motivation. Once the schedule is developed and agreed upon it may be helpful to hold a press conference to announce the programme to representatives of the media. Appendix G of Volume I provides samples of materials that can be used for such a press conference. Members of the local team should be given an opportunity to speak about the tasks they have undertaken.

23. Development of an Organizational Chart

The organizational chart should be presented graphically, and should indicate specific responsibilities and tasks as well as who reports to whom and how activities will be coordinated.

24. Preparation of Budget

Step One: Zero-budget exercise

The team should assume a zero-dollar budget – that is, discuss actions that can be taken using existing infrastructure and public communication tools (e.g. public service announcements; inclusion in existing in-service training for emergency room physicians; using speakers at professional meetings and conventions to reach groups of public health professionals).

The participants themselves need to determine what their participation will be and how they might best use their expertise and contacts in the community to help achieve the goals of the programme.

Step Two: Determination of baseline expense

In this step, the team should determine what expenses are absolutely necessary for initial, low-budget action items to initiate and maintain the programme.

Step Three: Determine budget

The team should then determine the price tag of other action items that are necessary to achieve the stated goals.

Step Four: Review of budget, goals and action plan

The team should review the available budget (in relation to the timetable and action plan) and determine how best to use available funds for leverage. For example, money might be invested in a campaign to generate additional funds from community action groups and local businesses. The team should also initiate fund-raising efforts. Suggestions for fund raising are provided in Volume I, Appendix H.

25. Official Recognition from WPA

At this point, the Action Team should submit the materials they have assembled in Steps 1–24 and a description of the way in which the project will be implemented to the WPA, and request recognition as an official participating site in the Worldwide Programme to Fight the Stigma and Discrimination because of Schizophrenia.

The proposal will then be considered for WPA sponsorship by the Steering Committee (during the trial phases of the programme) and by the Executive Committee (once the programme is released). Groups who would like to implement the programme without WPA Programme Sponsorship should also contact WPA to acknowledge that they are using material produced by WPA and inform WPA about the outcome of the programme.

The proposal should be sent to: Professor Norman Sartorius at the Département de Psychiatrie, 16–18 Bd de St Georges, 1205 Genève, Switzerland.

IV. Adaptation, development, pre-testing and revision of programme tools

Many of the steps described in the following section will be undertaken at the same time. For example, at the same time as the baseline survey is being done, the Action Team will also be reviewing the central theme and specific objectives of their programme in light of the results being obtained from the survey, deciding on the specific messages that will be central to the programme, evaluating existing media materials and determining which important messages are not included in the existing materials.

26. Baseline Survey

After the preceding determinations have been made, the Action Team should undertake a baseline survey to measure knowledge, attitudes and behaviour. This survey should be done at the same time as materials are being developed. Information gathered during this baseline measurement will help inform the media messages and ensure that the messages that are developed are relevant for the local community. The baseline survey will also provide data against which the outcomes of the programme can be measured (see Step 17).

27. Selection of Available Media Materials

Before embarking on the creation of new media materials, the team should thoroughly examine the existing available materials gathered in Step 15 to see if their stated messages and the media in which they were developed are appropriate for the programme. This will eliminate duplication of efforts, build upon the successes of previous programmes, and minimize cost.

28. Agreement on Central Theme and Programme Concepts

The Action Team should spend time at this point reviewing once again their understanding of the central theme and specific objectives of the programme, and considering whether the material they have found will be useful and usable in the programme.

29. Development of Message Concepts

The team should develop message concepts consisting of preliminary illustrations, words, phrases, and theme lines or slogans that reflect the overall strategy. These message concepts should be part of a single, unified campaign which will include common graphical and typographical elements, as well as a single theme that will continually reinforce the main concepts. Examples of thematic concepts that might be appropriate for selected target audiences are listed in Volume I, Appendix K.

Message concepts should be appropriate to the targeted audiences, relative to their needs and level of knowledge (e.g. information on medication side effects might not be appropriate for high school students, but would be for caregivers). Facts should be stated briefly in an easily comprehensible style. Messages that are ambiguous or require a great deal of explanation should be avoided. All messages should include a call-to-action. Phone numbers, addresses and other means of communication should be provided to allow the target audiences to respond.

In composing message concepts, the group should also think about how it will evaluate whether a message was effective; the formulation of outcome indicators can thus be linked to message development.

30. Decision on Production of New Materials

The team then needs to compile a list of message concepts that are central to the programme (see Step 29) and identify those concepts for which it has no communication materials (see Step 27). The team can then decide what new materials need to be produced and estimate the cost of such production.

31. Pre-test of Message Concepts

To achieve effective communication, it is crucial to test messages among audiences for whom they are intended before production. The opinions of experts, government officials or friends are not a sufficient guide to ensure effectiveness. Pre-testing and subsequent, often multiple, revisions of materials are as important to communication projects as evaluation and diagnosis are to the provision of health and mental health services.

It is recommended that the concepts be pre-tested with groups or individuals who are representative of the intended audiences to identify the concepts with the most potential. Give special attention to pictures or other non-verbal materials since these are easily misunderstood.

32. Development of Media Materials

The team should then convert concepts into complete messages and decide what media it will use for each message (e.g. radio announcements, booklets, posters).

In selecting the media it is important to carefully balance the goals of reach versus frequency. For example, television is an excellent medium for reaching large numbers of people with low cost per thousand (CPM), but it is not as effective as radio for generating greater frequency for the same cost per thousand. Professional meetings are excellent forums for reaching very targeted audiences. The possibility of measuring outcomes should also be considered in selecting media.

Volume I, Appendix K provides a list of factors to consider in developing media messages.

33. Pre-test of Materials

Complete messages and materials should be pre-tested for comprehension, recall, strong and weak points, personal relevance, and sensitive or controversial elements with representatives of the intended audiences before final production. Programme staff at all levels must be flexible and ready to make unanticipated changes as a result of testing.

34. Finalization of Communication Materials

After pre-testing the materials, the group should draw up a complete production schedule and media plan for the materials. The group should decide in what order the materials will be released to ensure a smooth flow of communication. For example, advertisements should not be released until follow-up materials are ready to be distributed to those who respond.

V. Implementation and monitoring of the programme

35. Building Local Support and Consensus Building

After materials have been pre-tested and are being prepared for distribution, a parallel effort to build consensus and support among influential members of the community should be conducted. This consensus building has a three-fold purpose:

- To ensure the formal approval of those who will help implement the programme in the community.
- To involve professionals and politicians who might not have been able to participate in the earlier planning process. These individuals should be shown clear evidence of the results expected in the community. If this presentation is done well, this effort should also enlist the help of new members who will assist in the implementation of the programme.

- To leverage the assistance of politicians in moving efforts from a local to a national level, and ultimately, to a global level.

36. Implementation of Programme by Local Action Team Members

While Step 35 is being conducted, the Local Action Team should:

- Schedule and integrate distribution of messages and materials through appropriate channels to maximize impact.
- Train those who will be using materials, as needed. For example, it is far preferable to have teachers attend a half-day symposium conducted by an expert in the field than to simply distribute teachers' guides. Speakers' bureaux operated by people with schizophrenia or their families have been successful in communicating with groups in the community. Such groups can benefit from training.

37. Coordination of Implementation Schedules with All Team Members

During meetings at this point, the team should decide on specific arrangements for implementing schedules and circulating reports so that no key personnel or group will be surprised by the appearance of any materials, and actions can be coordinated.

38. Maintenance of Programme Diary

The programme diary (introduced in Step 7) should be updated on a regular basis. This information will be essential during the evaluation phase and for future implementation of the programme both nationally and as part of the knowledge base of the global anti-stigma effort.

39. Monitoring

The group should compare project outputs with the original work plan and budget. This will help project leaders identify and correct problems before they become obstacles. Monitoring should cover:

- the volume of materials produced (e.g. quantities of brochures and newsletters printed);
- the distribution in media (e.g. ensuring advertising spots are run as agreed);
- the attendance at presentations and verifying that training sessions were conducted;
- the function of the teams, and adherence to work schedule and budget;
- the relationships with other agencies, including service providers and cooperating or hostile organizations;
- the quality of the products and process.

VI. Evaluation of the programme

40. Post-Test of Knowledge, Attitudes and Behaviour

The post-test should be formulated before the basic survey is conducted and there should be a correspondence between the two so that the effects of the programme can be evaluated (see Steps 16 and 17, and Volume I, Appendix D).

41. Evaluation of the Programme

Evaluation of the programme should examine the input (how much was invested), the process (what was done, what happened), the output (the effects of the intervention), the impact (effects on other areas or actions) and outcome (an overall evaluation of the process and its effects in relation to the broad goals of the programme).

Be sure to consider this final checklist:

• Are you reaching your full target audiences?
• Are you reaching your target audiences with enough exposures to ensure that your message is noted, recognized and remembered?
• What is the final budget, including media production and placement (see Step 24)?
• Is this budget adequate to meet the originally stated goals?

An example of a stigma-reduction intervention in London provides an illustration of how these five levels of evaluation are applied. In this intervention (Wolff, 1997), neighbours of a new group home for people with mental illness in South London were canvassed door-to-door and provided with educational materials about mental illness, including videotapes and written materials. Social events were also organized. This programme was then evaluated using the following criteria:

Input: Production of videotapes, written materials, discussion sessions.
Process: Did neighbours view videotapes and read brochures?
Output: Did neighbours' fearful and rejecting attitudes decrease?
Impact: Did neighbours make friends with patients?
Outcome: Did patients have a better quality of life as a result? Did the community accept the patients and was it satisfied with its decision? (In fact, 13% of neighbours made friends with patients or invited them into their homes.)

42. Review of Overall Outcomes

The overall outcome of the programme should be reviewed and the findings described in order to plan for future activities or assist planning at other sites. The team should recall overall and short-term objectives at this stage and examine the programme diary as well as other written materials developed in the programme.

The Local Action Team should conduct the analysis jointly. This analysis should include the following.

Review and analysis of each stage of programme

This step should be done to evaluate the work in each step of the programme. This will allow the groups in other sites to learn from the experience of others.

Analysis of effect on proposed audiences and broader community

Was the intended outcome achieved? Were there other, unintended results of the programme?

Analysis of media effectiveness

The group should evaluate the effectiveness of the media they selected. There are many methods that can be used to assess media selection (see Volume I, Appendix F).

Changes in the system

In addition to assessing whether the objectives have been reached, the team should consider the following:

- *Changes in the legal system*. Were laws protecting the rights of psychiatric patients enacted? Were new laws drafted?
- *Changes in portrayal of people with schizophrenia in the media*. Were fewer people with schizophrenia portrayed as villains in television shows or movies? Have there been more news stories that stress the importance of early diagnosis or the importance of reintegrating those with schizophrenia back into society?
- *Changes in employment of those with schizophrenia*. Have employment figures for those with schizophrenia increased?
- *Changes in support for families*. Has there been an increase in the number of support programmes for families?
- *Changes in funding*. Has the amount of the government's financial support for mental health care increased?
- *Changes in government's administrative structure*. Have there been changes in administrative bodies (e.g. appointment of an official specifically concerned with patient rights?

Changes in national environment

If the programme was done only in a part of the country, have there been changes in national environment? Did news of these local efforts reach other areas of the country and influence others on a broader scale?

Identification of strengths and weaknesses

This section should provide specific examples and hindsight wisdom.

Evaluation of skills acquired by local personnel

Has training produced long-term benefits among individuals who interact with those with schizophrenia, such as law enforcement officials and emergency room personnel? Would some of these individuals be useful as trainers in the future?

Examination of linkage to other mental health and health care initiatives locally and nationally

Are there ways we can disseminate successful interventions to other areas, such as providing high school teaching materials to teachers over a broader area?

VII. Planning action after programme ends

43. Assuring continuation of work after the End of the Programme

The group should now look for additional sources of financial support both to extend the current programme and to implement additional initiatives. It should also attempt to enforce and support networks that have been created and provide active participants with ideas on support in the future.

44. Documenting the Project

A meeting or press conference should be held to disseminate results and recommendations to all those who participated in the project. Such an event would also allow those who have heard of the programme's success to learn more and become involved in the ongoing effort.

A written summary of the process steps undertaken in the action programme and an account of outcome should be produced, and could be written up in a manner that will facilitate its widespread use. A specific report should also be provided to the WPA for use in further dissemination of the model around the world. Efforts should be made to publish the results of the programme in well-read scientific journals.

45. Replanning for Future Development (applying the lessons)

Can lessons learned from the project be applied to future stigma-reducing activities? What results of the assessment should be incorporated into the programme design?

REFERENCE

Wolff, G. (1997). Attitudes of the media and the public. In: Leff, J., ed. *Care in the Community: Illusion or Reality?* Wiley, New York.

Appendices to Volume I

Appendix A

Instructions for conducting a site survey

The purpose of the site survey is not epidemiological; rather the goal is to get a clearer idea of the characteristics of the site so that programme efforts can be effectively targeted. It is therefore important not to spend an excessive amount of time on the survey nor allow it to become too detailed.

Who conducts the survey?

The Local Action Team may first want to determine which of its professional members have experience in developing such research tools. The group may also decide that they want to engage the services of an outside research agency. Care should be taken that the survey is done in a way that can be repeated so that the effectiveness of the programme can be clearly measured during the assessment phase.

Who and what is surveyed?

There is, of course, often a trade-off between the completeness of the information gathered, and time and budget considerations. However, the survey should aim to give a clear picture of the community's knowledge, attitudes and behaviour to guide action, and allow measurement of results. The survey should determine both:

• What is the stigma and discrimination because of schizophrenia now (see Part II of Volume 2 for a detailed discussion of the origins and extent of stigma and discrimination)?
• What knowledge, attitudes and behaviour should be changed? The survey should be broader than the intended action, since the efforts of the project may have an impact in areas unanticipated during the planning process. For example, while teachers and high school students may be part of the identified target audiences, our messages will also reach the parents and siblings of these students and other members of the general public, whose behaviour may change as a consequence.

Information that should be obtained

(a) Demographics
- Age and sex. The distribution of the population of the site by age and sex should be ascertained, using the age groups: 0–15 years; 16–29 years; 30–65 years; 66+ years.

(b) Education
- Structure of the educational system.
- Proportion of the population in school (at all levels).
- Differences/profile of those in various levels of school.
- Methods for communicating with teachers and administrators.
- Social class distinctions in the educational system.
- Literacy rates.

(c) Economic features
- What percentage of people live under the poverty line?
- How important is the barter economy?
- What is the geographical distribution of economic resources?
- What are the main sources of income for the population?
- What is the level of unemployment?
- What percentage of the population is employed by others?

(d) Geography
- What is the geographical distribution of the community (e.g. urban versus rural dispersion)?
- What are the climate and topography of the region and how do they affect accessibility (i.e. are all areas equally accessible to health services and media year round)?

(e) Social characteristics
The team should identify opportunities for and impediments to communications, including:

- Is the community socially cohesive?
- Are there festivals or gatherings providing opportunities for communication?
- Are there social networks in place for communication and action?
- Does the community provide support for the poor and indigent? If so, what type of support is provided?
- Do NGOs or social action groups exist in the community?
- What consumer and family groups exist in the community?
- Are there religious and/or business organizations that can create events and opportunities for socializing and communicating?

- What is the predominant family size/profile (e.g. single-parent households)?
- What are the patterns of drug and alcohol use in the area?
- What are the crime rates in the area? Are there significant differences between areas (e.g. parts of the town) in these or other respects?

(f) Cultural characteristics

The team should consider questions about the cultural beliefs and customs of the site that may affect the outcome of the programme, including:

- What are the common cultural conceptions about the causes of mental illness?
- What are the prevailing political and religious ideologies concerning causes of mental illness?
- Who is generally believed to be responsible for giving help and support to the disabled?
- Do traditional healers or practitioners of alternative medicine have an important role in the treatment of mental illness?
- What are the cultural norms concerning social behaviour (e.g. is someone who does not work and earn his own living not a fully accepted member of society, or is there tolerance towards people who are dependent on others for their needs)?
- What is the prevailing family system – intergenerational or a preponderance of one-generation or single-household families?
- Is the area largely industrial and urban, or rural and agricultural?
- Do rural families in the area provide care for their disabled members?
- How important a role do religion and churches play in the culture and society of the area?
- *Are the charitable activities of local churches limited to their members or do they reach a wider population?*

(g) Attitudes towards people with schizophrenia

Are results available from studies on attitudes relative to mental health in general and schizophrenia in particular?

It may be necessary to carry out an informal mini-survey of the attitudes of particular groups within a community. Such a survey might include:

- small focus groups;
- visits to prisons;
- discussions with legislators;
- an analysis of newspaper reporting of mental health issues over a year in widely read journals;
- attitudes of medical students;
- an anthropological survey of folklore relative to mental health issues;

- letters to various users of psychiatric services and their relatives asking for instances in which they have experienced discrimination.

Since attitudes may vary from one social group to another, it will be necessary to evaluate attitudes on a group-by-group basis according to a distribution of groups that is relevant to the particular community.

Appendix B

Survey of national health/mental health policies and services

The team needs to gather baseline data on the health and mental health policies and services of the site. In gathering this information, the team should consult legislators, local social services offices, hospital administrators and directors, and representatives of the insurance industry. The main questions to be considered are:

- What are the main features of the mental health treatment system?
- Which are the responsible authorities at local, regional and national levels?
- What are the methods of financing and organizing services (i.e. who pays for mental health care)?
- What is the insurance structure?
- Are equal benefits provided for mental health treatment as for other medical conditions? If not, which areas are particularly unequal?
- Is disability aid available?
- Who provides formal care for persons with mental disorders (i.e. professions involved)?
- Are there any population groups that are currently not receiving care or for whom care is inadequate?
- How many psychiatrists practise in the area and how are they organized?
- What training in psychiatry is given: For psychiatrists? General medical students?
- Is there some in-service training in general for psychiatry?
- How many general practitioners are in the area?
- How many homes for the elderly are in the area and how are they organized?
- What is total number of beds used for psychiatric care in the community?
- How many people with schizophrenia are in institutions (including inpatient hospital facilities, nursing homes, residential facilities, etc.)?
- Are patients with psychiatric illnesses frequently treated in facilities outside the site area?
- What access to care do families of those with schizophrenia have?
- Is homelessness a problem? If so, are any measures taken to help the homeless?
- What services are available: Outpatient? Inpatient? Transitional? Rehabilitation?

- How are inpatient and outpatient resources allocated?
- Do institutions dealing with mental disorders provide patients with opportunities for vocational training?
- Are there sheltered workshops that will employ people diagnosed as having a mental illness or impairment? Is there a waiting list? If so, how long is that list?
- Do working relationships exist between the mental health service and other health services? If so, how close are these alliances?
- How much do those working in the health care system know about schizophrenia?
- What laws and legal practices regarding the care, treatment and confinement of people with schizophrenia are used in the area?
- Is there involuntary treatment? Confinement?
- What rights/protections are in place for people with schizophrenia?
- What are the circumstances surrounding people with schizophrenia who are in jail, prison or who have committed crimes?
- Can they (and do they) receive treatment while in penal institutions?

Appendix C

Survey of communication resources

It is important to obtain information about communication opportunities. For example, in rural areas (if these are to be included), there may be fewer television or radios per capita. The following information should be gathered to identify available media and communication resources:

- names of editors and medical columnists of local newspapers;
- executives and directors of local radio and television stations;
- number and proportion of households with television;
- number and proportion of households with radios;
- media most frequently accessed by various target groups in the site area;
- radio and television networks;
- private and public channels and stations;
- provisions for broadcasting public service announcements;
- most accessible channels and stations;
- percentage of country covered by different channels/stations;
- broadcast languages used;
- proportion of local versus imported programming;
- proportion of automobiles with radios;
- videocassette recorder (VCR) penetration;
- satellite penetration;

- print media;
- national daily newspapers and their circulation;
- consumer magazines and their circulation;
- comic books sold;
- other popular media;
- attitude to foreign media;
- influence of foreign media and media from neighbouring areas.

Appendix D

Recommendations for outcome measures

Introduction

Project assessments should be undertaken in terms of realistic measurable outcomes which are spelt out in the project objectives. These can be seen as a continuum affecting knowledge, attitudes and behaviour of members of the target audiences, including service providers and influential groups. Outcome assessment steps include:

- measure and track audience' awareness, recognition, comprehension, recall and practice using appropriate and affordable research techniques to obtain rapid feedback;
- analyse results in terms of specific objectives;
- make necessary revisions in project design.

Outcome measures will have to be designed locally, at least in part. The basis for this formulation will be the listing of examples of discrimination by the Local Action Group and the ranking of the challenges in the daily life of people living with schizophrenia and their families. The Local Action Group will need to record changes in the lives of these individuals that have most probably been related to the programme.

In addition to measuring outcomes based on these indicators, it will also be necessary to assess success in changing some of the processes underlying discrimination. The list given in this appendix presents suggestions in this regard. The Local Action Group should rate these suggestions from most to least relevant and then assess the difficulty of obtaining the necessary information at the site.

Overall goals

- To increase knowledge and understanding of schizophrenia among the general public, key community figures and policy-makers.

- To improve the social acceptance and community integration of people with schizophrenia.

Recommendation

Each subcommittee of the project should develop its own overall goals and some examples of measurable objectives. Below, we list goals and some possible objectives for the anti-stigma group. Each subcommittee's list of goals and objectives should be sent to the group chairman.

Examples of measurable goals

To increase knowledge among the general public concerning the causes of schizophrenia.
Measure: Knowledge survey of the general public.

To increase the awareness of the general public that schizophrenia can be episodic and treatable.
Measure: Telephone survey of the general public.

To decrease by X% the number of people who perceive people with schizophrenia as violent.
Measure: Survey of the general public.

To change judicial attitudes regarding people with schizophrenia and law enforcement.
Measure: Attitude survey of police, attorneys and judges.

To increase the number of decision-makers using person-first language (referring to 'people with schizophrenia').
Measure: Text analysis of policy documents and articles in the media.

To increase education in high schools about schizophrenia.
Measure: Survey of recent teaching practice of high school health and science teachers. Knowledge survey of high school students.

To increase discussion of schizophrenia among the general public.
Measure: Content analysis of popular media articles.

To increase the access of people with schizophrenia to social resources.
Measure: Survey of social agencies (subsidized housing, vocational services, etc.) to assess proportion of recipients who are people with schizophrenia.

To reduce the number of people with schizophrenia in jail.
Measure: Survey of local jail population.

To increase the general public's active tolerance for people with schizophrenia.
Measure: Survey of sample of people with schizophrenia to assess: proportion employed, length of residence in current accommodation and the

number of work schemes that bring patients into contact with the general public.

To develop a local anti-stigma advocacy ('stigma-busters') group at each site.
Measures: A stigma-buster group has been established; has been in existence for 6 months and has achieved a success.

To establish a consumer speakers' bureau at each site.
Measures: A speakers' bureau has been established; has been in existence for 6 months and has given X presentations.

To increase by X% the number of employers who hire people with schizophrenia.
Measure: Employer survey.

Appendix E

Examples of the kinds of stigma and discrimination that occur because of schizophrenia

Stigma and discrimination because of schizophrenia can take many forms. It is important to obtain local accounts in each of the programme sites of ways in which stigma is expressed, as well as the ways and places in which discrimination occurred.

In producing this account, the Local Action Group should rely upon information obtained from patients and their relatives. Human Rights activists should also be consulted.

Health care workers (including psychiatrists, family physicians and social workers) should also be consulted, particularly those who practice in the community and are in regular contact with patients. Observations from social scientists should be taken into account, particularly if they have been active in this area (e.g. dealing with the plight of the homeless). Theoretical and overly general formulations should be avoided and an inductive method, beginning with the personal experiences of those most concerned, is recommended.

In considering stigma and discrimination, the Local Action Group should be aware that positive as well as negative stigma and discrimination should be recorded. An example of positive discrimination might be the protection of people with schizophrenia from losing their employment when an industrial plant is downsized.

Discrimination based on fact should be distinguished from discrimination based on prejudice and various false beliefs.

Appendix F

Advantages and disadvantages of various media

Slides/binders

Advantages
- Relatively low cost.
- User familiarity with the technology.

Disadvantages
- Dependent on slide projector and presentation environment.
- Less uniformity of presentation.
- Dependent on availability of knowledgeable presenter.

Brochures (16 to 24 pages)

Advantages
- Can be shipped virtually anywhere.
- Low-to-moderate cost.

Disadvantages
- Limited amount of information content.
- Language dependent.
- Likely to be disregarded unless content is very distinctive.

Pamphlets/books (36+ pages)

Advantages
- Comprehensive information with more space for case histories.
- Access–quality publication will be retained on bookshelf.

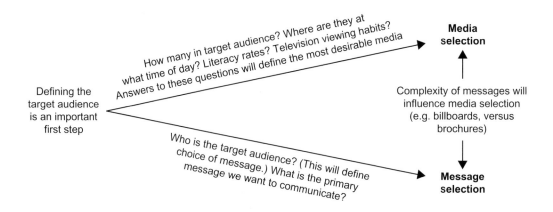

Figure A2.

Disadvantages
- One person, one book.
- Static presentation.

Comic books
Advantages
- Popular and widely read in some countries.
- Of particular interest with larger populations of lower socio-economic classes.

Disadvantages
- A challenge to produce so that the message is creatively and effectively embedded in a popular story.
- Culture specific, idiom dependent.

Audiotapes
Advantages
- The verisimilitude and emotional power of audio.
- A controlled presentation.

Disadvantages
- No visuals (or limited to explanatory companion brochure).
- Linear format, does not lend itself to quick access.

Films/Videos
Advantages
- High visual content for even greater verisimilitude and emotional impact.
- Higher learning with greater sense stimulus.

Disadvantages
- Dependent on variety of videotape technologies.
- Language barriers (overdubbing or subtitle).

Multimedia
Advantages
- Near encyclopedic content with easy access to necessary information.
- Synergies of video, text and sound with multiple language capability.
- Active participation versus passive learning.

Disadvantages
- Dependent on personal computer availability.
- Relatively higher cost for fully realized video input.

Web sites

Advantages
- Zero postage for distribution of materials.
- Readily lends itself to constant updating and active data gathering.

Disadvantages
- Dependent on computer and phone lines.
- Information content may be limited.
- Reaches a limited group of the population.

Teleconferences

Advantages
- A national or worldwide event.
- High visibility for conference participants.

Disadvantages
- A one-time event.
- Highly dependent on logistics for presenters and viewers.
- Logistical problems of immediate translation.

Media matrix

	Reach	Information content	Language dependence	Retention/ repetition	Capital investment
Slides/binders	Moderate	Low to Moderate	Moderate	Low	Low
Brochures	High	Moderate	Moderate	Moderate	Low to Moderate
Pamphlets/ books	High	High	Low to Moderate	Moderate to High	Moderate to High
Audiotapes	Moderate	Moderate	Moderate	Low to Moderate	Moderate
Films Videos	Moderate	Moderate	Moderate	Moderate	Moderate to High
Multimedia	Moderate	High	Moderate	High	Moderate to High
Web sites	Moderate	Moderate	Moderate to High	Moderate to High	Moderate
Teleconferences	Low	Low	Moderate to High	Low	High

Reach is defined as the number of people who will receive and be able to use the materials based on technological (not language) considerations.

Information content is defined as the amount of information that will 'fit' in a particular medium.

Language dependence is defined as the degree to which the programme depends on a written or spoken language.

Retention/repetition is defined as the ability to re-visit the information and the ability to retrieve a particular piece of information (e.g. the linear nature of audio-tapes is more limited than printed material in which one can 'turn to' a particular piece of information).

In addition to this overview of media, media buying agencies can also supply comparative information that will better enable you to evaluate particular media for a particular target group.

It will be important to connect local communication experts and discuss the above table to decide on the media to be used. Their comments as well as experience with media on the local level should be recorded. Some forms of communication are not included in this chart. These should be added wherever possible (e.g. comic books, folk songs, theatres, puppet theatres, plays and playactings.)

The variety of measures that can be used to evaluate communication effectiveness is almost as great as the number of communication firms who conduct such evaluations. We give just a few examples of the kinds of measures that can be used to evaluate one medium in comparison with others. Certain qualitative measures can take into consideration the media vehicle's audience size adjusted by a scale of values reflecting:

- audience' characteristics in relation to a segmental (targeted) strategy;
- intermedia differences;
- intramedia differences;
- advertising unit differences.

Gench (1970) defined five factors to consider in measuring the effectiveness of a media vehicle:

1 *Editorial climate:* the authority or believability of the publication.
2 *Message fit:* the appropriateness of the message to the medium and target audiences.
3 *Technical capabilities:* a qualitative measure of a particular vehicle in comparison with others in the medium (e.g. clarity of the frequency modulation (FM) over the amplitude modulation (AM) signal in certain geographical regions).
4 *Competing messages:* presence of other advertisements for the same or similar advertisers that may add to confusion and message clutter.
5 *Target population receptiveness:* Gench comments 'The social context in which a media vehicle is viewed or read can make a difference. Some communication may be intended to reach the entire family as a group. Thus, evening television would be more desirable than daytime television, magazines or newspapers.'

REFERENCE – APPENDIX F

Gench, D.H. (1970). Media factors: a review article. *Journal of Marketing Research*, **7**, 216–225.

Appendix G

Creating a press event

1. News conferences

The news conference is an opportunity to provide timely, relevant and important information to the media. It is important that your message or event be of major importance. A mistake many communications teams make is the overuse of the news conference, which will only result in journalists and media representatives coming to view subsequent press events (which may, in fact, be more newsworthy) with scepticism.

Speakers should be chosen carefully. Two speakers will provide a focus for attendees, with other sources available to the press for comment after the conference. A notable person with credentials upon whom the press can rely for reliable information will increase attendance and coverage.

The conference should be limited to 30–40 min with at least 20 min allotted for questions. Speakers should be available to the press for individual comment after the conference itself.

The following guidelines based on experience in the US, Canada and some European countries may help you organize a successful press conference:

- Schedule your news conference for mid-morning. This allows reporters time to meet afternoon deadlines.
- Choose a familiar site that is centrally located in your community to hold your conference. Or choose a prestigious setting that is relevant to your event/message.
- A Tuesday, Wednesday or Thursday is the best day to schedule a press conference.
- If your news conference allows for advance notice to the press, send out media advisories 1 week prior to the event. Always include the address of a contact person and a phone number for more information.
- If your news conference is being held in response to a breaking event or news, your issue will be of major significance to the media. If you do not receive a significant amount of interest from the media (in the form of some verbal acknowledgement from representatives of both print and broadcast media), you should reconsider holding the press event.
- Use your local news advisory services. In many countries, the wire services run listings of news events so that the press can determine what to cover. Find out the

deadline for inclusion in the Daybook and send written notice to the Daybook Editor prior to the deadline. (A Daybook is a document that is updated daily and lists new stories that are being considered.)

- Hire a photographer to cover the event. Many local publications will be unable to send a photographer, so your ability to provide the reporter with a photograph will improve the reporting and your relationship with the reporter.
- Provide press kits. Press kits should include fact sheets and background information about schizophrenia. Also provide a copy of the prepared remarks of the speakers. Include biographies of your speakers in the press kits.
- Prepare your speakers for dealing with the media. Give each speaker a time limit for his or her remarks. Hold a mock press conference to practice and ask the speakers questions you believe are likely to arise. Rehearsal is very important. Schedule time for it.
- Make follow-up phone calls to the press (1–2 days in advance for newspaper editors, 1 day for radio news directors and the same day for television assignment editors), since television schedules change frequently.
- The venue for the press conference should be large enough to accommodate all press and camera crews. The room should have good lighting, even though most camera crews will bring additional lights. Position the podium or head table to allow an unobstructed view from anywhere in the room. Chairs should be arranged to provide the media with a clear view of the podium or head table. Supply a remote box for multiple sound output for recording devices. Arrive at the site at least 1 h in advance to make sure every last detail has been arranged.
- Have a press registration table complete with sign-in sheets and press kits, which will allow you to survey the media attendance for the conference, further cultivate your relationships with the press, and enhance your ability to follow up with reporters after the conference.
- Provide refreshments for the press, especially if the conference is mid-morning.
- Start your news conference on time and end it when scheduled. Reporters have very tight schedules and you can damage your reputation with representatives of the press by not being punctual or letting your speakers talk too long.

Note: As mentioned above, if you cannot gather enough attendees together for the press conference or if the announcement is an update of information previously released, you may want to send a press kit to appropriate editors in the print and broadcast media.

The press kit

Press kits should be compiled for specific events or to provide background information about schizophrenia and the relevance of the announcement to be made.

Prepare extra kits and keep them on file to send to reporters who request additional information. (A sample is included in the media toolkit and a list of contents is given below.) The press kits should include:

- news release (for specific event);
- fact sheets on schizophrenia (usually one to two pages): focus on key points concerning the personal and social impact of the stigma of schizophrenia;
- the programme's goals and objectives;
- background information on the WPA and the organizations involved in your local effort;
- brochures, newsletters and other outreach materials;
- questions and answers document to answer some of the commonly asked questions about schizophrenia and the stigma surrounding it;
- resource materials might also include articles about schizophrenia, information on your Local Action Group or speeches given by someone in your group.

The media kit folder is usually a two-pocket folder, which has the news release on the right-hand side to ensure visibility. All materials should carry a date of printing at the bottom of the last page to avoid old releases being picked up and rerun.

The news release

The news release is intended to focus on the key aspects of your story. It should be limited to two or three double-spaced pages. Other documentation will provide technical or additional reference materials; the news release should be very much targeted to the announcement of the day.

When reviewing a news release, editors treat it as an inverted pyramid; generally they begin cutting from the bottom up to fit the information into the format. Therefore, the first paragraph should contain the main ideas of the story, with each subsequent paragraph elaborating on the key information in the first paragraph.

Content of the release

It is important to try to answer the following six basic questions as well as providing a news hook (with some local relevance to the reader) in the first paragraph:

- WHO (is involved, or to whom did it happen).
- WHAT (was said or done; or what is going to happen).
- WHEN (did or will the story or event take place).
- WHERE (did it happen, where will it take place).
- WHY (did it happen or will it happen).
- HOW (did it happen or will it happen).

Tips for writing the news release

- Always type your release, double-spaced.
- In the upper left-hand side of the release, type 'FOR IMMEDIATE RELEASE'; or if the release time and date is specific, indicate the release date.
- Keep the headline of the release short (10 words or less) and TYPE IT IN ALL UPPER CASE. The headline should let the reader know exactly what the press release is about and its relevance/importance to the reader.
- The body of the text of the release should begin with the city where the event or conference is being held (e.g. Geneva, 2 January, 19__).
- Limit your release to no more than four pages. Number each page. At the bottom of each page (if additional ages are listed), type 'MORE'. On the last page of the release, type '###' or '-30-' to indicate the end.
- Do not split a sentence between pages.
- Include approved quotes from authorities on the issue in your release.
- If you use abbreviations or acronyms of any kind, be sure to spell out the full name, title or phrase (e.g. World Psychiatric Association [WPA]).
- Your press release should end with the name and phone number of a key contact person who can answer questions.

Follow-up

Whether you have held a full news conference or have sent out a press kit to editors and reporters, follow-up is key. Out of respect for their time, keep your follow-up call brief. Ask if any more information is needed and what kind of coverage may be expected.

Appendix H

Fund-raising guidelines

Obtaining funding for printed materials, seminars and other expenditures in a public communication campaign is a challenge. Ultimately, proper funding can make or break a programme.

Several guidelines are important to keep in mind as you develop a fund-raising programme:

- Develop a clearly defined goal. The more specific the request (e.g. raising money for a specific seminar or educational programme), the more likely you are to receive a positive response.
- Set a specific monetary goal. Estimate all costs in your programme so that you can give potential donors a clear understanding of your ultimate target.

- Identify in-house resources. Are there members of your Local Advisory Group who have access to funding?
- Develop a list of potential outside resources.
- Consider the following options (depending on local restrictions in the donation of money, your programme options may be more limited than those listed below):

  - *Annual campaigns*, so that potential donors can plan their giving in advance.
  - *Planned giving programmes*. This term is used to describe pre-planned forms of donation such as wills and bequests (often as a per cent of the estate of the donor).
  - *Pooled income funds* (a trust agreement in which money is transferred to the organization's pooled income fund directly).
  - *Trusts*: some individuals may choose to make your programme the beneficiary of a life insurance policy which will transfer funds on the owner's death.

- Your programme may use some of the following fund-raising strategies:

  - *Personal solicitations*: members of your group may approach individuals on a one-on-one basis.
  - *Direct mail*: this will allow you to reach a larger number of potential donors, although less personally. (The fund-raising letter is particularly important. It should get directly to the point and present a clear plan of action.)
  - *Telemarketing*: like direct mail, this allows you to reach a broad number of people with the added benefit of a phone conversation. However, it may be more difficult to reach people as directly as mail. Calls will also need to be repeated.
  - *Special sponsored events*: these can include awards programmes or dinners that might include a 'silent auction' for donated materials.

The solicitation package

Material should be prepared for individuals considering a contribution. The package should clearly explain:

- the goals of your fund-raising campaign;
- why your programme is important;
- the specific benefit the donor will receive (e.g. publicity);
- the effectiveness of your organization;
- several options for support or participation;
- the long-term value of the programme.

Follow these guidelines for writing the solicitation letter:

- Keep the letter to one page.
- Use clear concise language.

- Use letterhead with the organization's main phone number.
- Address letters to the appropriate person. Do *not* write 'Dear Sir or Madam'.
- Capture the reader's attention in the first sentence. State project goals in the first paragraph.
- Outline only the highlights of your request. Details may be covered in the proposal itself or discussed at a future meeting.
- Show how your programme addresses key concerns for the reader.

Along with the letter, you should provide: a prospectus summarizing the project, support and informational materials on schizophrenia, and a donor request card the donor can fill out and return.

Corporate recognition

Corporations and foundations often respond well when their company achieves greater visibility from the donation. A 'Corporate Giving Plan' establishes tiers of potential donations and might be constructed this way:

- Corporate Sponsor: $15,000 and higher.
- Corporate Benefactor: $10,000–15,000.
- Corporate Patron: $5000–10,000.
- Corporate Donor: $2500–5000.
- Corporate Contributor: up to $2500.

Appendix I

Baseline survey of knowledge, attitudes and behaviours

A variety of methods can be used to obtain information about knowledge and attitudes as well as some reports on behaviour. The three cheapest methods are mail surveys, telephone interviews and focus group interviews. Other types of surveys, such as house-to-house surveys with personal interviews, are less economically feasible. The following matrix provides an overview of the general advantages and disadvantages of different research methods:

Measurement consideration	Mail survey	Telephone interview	Focus group
Population	Allows you to approach larger numbers of people but with a one-time opportunity for response.	Allows you to reach a broader population but often requires repeated call-backs.	For smaller, more well-defined groups.

(continued)

Measurement consideration	Mail survey	Telephone interview	Focus group
Biased response*	Can be segmented geographically.	Allows for random dialling.	Some small group bias.
Item construction	Must be carefully worded, since there is no opportunity to clarify responses to questions.	Interviewers can clarify questions; open-ended questions are allowed.	Generally open-ended to facilitate open discussion.
Costs	Low per-person cost.	Modest per-person cost.	Higher per-person cost.
Speed	Responses arrive within 1–2 weeks; analysis of written questionnaires takes additional time.	Dependent on number of interviewers; analysis will take additional time.	Responses are immediate, but analysis of qualitative data can take considerable time.

*Biased response refers to how data might be segmented (perhaps a positive characteristic for your research) or skewed (the negative, limiting nature of the methods). For example, focus groups allow for more open qualitative exploration of issues but may be biased by interpersonal dynamics between participants.

Appendix J

Thematic concepts and sample messages

The team will need to select a single, unified theme for the programme, as well as specific messages related to that theme that target selected audiences. In this appendix, we present a number of thematic concepts that might be chosen as well as samples of targeted messages related to those concepts. Here are some examples:

Theme: Schizophrenia. The one thing IS it is treatable.

Message to general practitioners: Effective treatments for schizophrenia are available that have far fewer side effects than older medications.

Messages to teachers:

- Schizophrenia can be treated effectively. People can regain their ability to function in society.
- Schizophrenia is a biological illness that can be treated.
- Students need to learn to be tolerant and helpful towards those who are different.

- Students should be taught not to laugh at or ridicule those who are different.

Theme: Schizophrenia. Open the Doors.

- *Sample messages to police*:
- Bizarre or abnormal behaviour may be a symptom of mental illness.
- When you see someone who is behaving very oddly, consider having a doctor evaluate them or take them to the emergency room, but not to jail.

Theme: Schizophrenia. Look closer; you'll see the human being.

Appendix K

Factors to consider in developing media messages

Once the team has decided what messages need to be communicated to the target audiences, a media plan can be developed to determine the most effective media to select to achieve the stated goals. The following general measures can be used to select one medium over another (Sissors, 1997):

- optimum number of prospects;
- optimum amount of frequency;
- lowest cost per thousand (CPM);
- minimum waste (non-prospects);
- within the specified budget.

Traditional measurements of a particular vehicle's effectiveness (e.g. gross rating points or Neilsen ratings for television) can be helpful. However, when messages are being placed on a pro-bono or discounted rate, trade-offs are to be expected. For example, print ads may appear at the back of a magazine or television ads may be aired late in the evening well after prime time viewing hours. While the cost is attractive, your message will reach a more limited viewership. *For example of messages developed for the anti-stigma campaign, consult the Media Toolkit available from the WPA.*

In creating the actual messages, the team should consider some of the maxims and tips that copywriters and graphical designers have developed for the creation of ads. For example, Russell and Lane (1996) outlined the following principles for creating effective headlines in print advertising:

- use short simple words (usually no more than 10 words);
- include an invitation to the prospect to become involved;
- use an action verb;

- give enough information in the headline so that the prospect who reads it learns something.

Russell and Lane give the following guidelines for reviewing advertising copy:

- Develop a copy strategy: what to say and to whom.
- Does the message position the problem and its solution clearly?
- Does the message promise a benefit for the prospect?
- Does the message tie to the overall strategy?
- How strong is the execution of the 'big' idea? Is it bold and unexpected? Is it visually arresting? Is it single-minded?

Kaatz (1995) presents a checklist that the team can use to review the messages it has developed:

- Have you learnt everything you can about the problem and solution, or service, offered?
- Have you clearly defined your target audiences and their needs?
- Have you written to your target audiences as you would to a real-life person and not a research statistic?
- Have you promised a real benefit and backed it up with a reason why the person will receive this benefit?
- Have you recognized that the prospect's time is valuable by getting right to the point?
- Have you made certain that what you said relates to your unique challenge and cannot be easily transferred to another?
- Have you avoided saying more than necessary?
- Have you written with excitement and enthusiasm so your prospects will say: 'They really believe in what they are saying'?
- Have you rewarded your prospect by making it easy and fun to take time with your message?
- Have you remembered that the message is the centre of the advertisement, and not the advertisement itself?

REFERENCES – APPENDIX K

Kaatz, R. (1995). *Advertising and Marketing Checklists*, 2nd edn. NTC Business Books.

Russell, J., Lane, W.R. (1996). *Kleppner's Advertising Procedure*, 13th edn. Prentice Hall Press, pp. 516–517.

Sissors, J. (1997). *Advertising Media Planning*. NTC Business Books.

Appendix II
Decreasing stigma

(Note: The following is an excerpt from Volume II of the programme materials. The full volume is available electronically and can be downloaded at www.openthedoors.com/english/01-02.html)

What are stigma, prejudice, and discrimination?

The word 'stigma' is of Greek origin and means 'to pierce, to make a hole.' The word was also used, however, to mean branding a criminal with a hot iron to mark infamy. In the Anatomy of Melancholy, Burton spoke of being 'stigmatized with hot iron.' It was in the late middle ages that the word came to mean the public defaming and branding of a criminal so that all could recognize him. Other meanings of the word, in particular with reference to stigmata (wounds similar to those of Christ indicating that a person has lived a life of extraordinary sanctity), have gradually disappeared. In more recent years, stigma has been used especially to indicate that certain diagnoses (e.g. tuberculosis, cancer and mental illness) awaken prejudice against persons so diagnosed.

Prejudice is an attitude reflecting the readiness of people to act in a positive or negative way towards the object of the prejudice without examining whether there is any justification for such behaviour. There are numerous prerequisites for prejudice to develop. Several of the most important are:

- *Recognition of the object of prejudice*: for example, prejudice is awakened once the individual admits that he has a mental disorder or when extra pyramidal side-effects make it clear to others that he has been receiving anti-psychotic medication.
- *Social acceptance of the prejudice*: there is an absence of any strong reaction by others to the prejudice.
- *Lack of personal knowledge about the object of prejudice*: for example, serving in the same military unit with people from a different race can help reduce prejudice against those belonging to that racial group.

The literature concerning breaking down prejudice indicates that there are numerous methods of eliminating or weakening prejudice, but that none of them is easy or quick.

Discrimination is a particularly negative consequence of stigma and prejudice. It means that individuals or groups in a society deprive others of rights or benefits because of stigma and prejudice. For example, those given a diagnosis of schizophrenia are often denied the rights or benefits they would have if they were not given such a diagnosis. Discrimination because of schizophrenia is expressed in numerous ways, including lack of parity in reimbursement for care, injustice in legislation, unwillingness to employ people with schizophrenia and refusal to allow someone with a mental disorder entry into a social group (e.g. by way of marriage). In terms of priorities, there is no doubt that discrimination should be the first target of action – not only because it is the most direct form of harm inflicted on those with mental illness, but also because the reducing discrimination (e.g. in the laws) in turn helps reduce stigma and consequent prejudice.

What is the stigma because of schizophrenia?

The general public and even health professionals tend to hold a stereo-typed image of those with schizophrenia. This image usually involves some or all of the following misconceptions:

- Nobody recovers from schizophrenia.
- Schizophrenia is an untreatable disease.
- People with schizophrenia are usually violent and dangerous.
- People with schizophrenia are likely to infect others with their madness.
- People with schizophrenia are lazy and unreliable.
- Schizophrenia is the result of a deliberate weakness of will and character ('the person could snap out of it if he wanted').
- Everything people with schizophrenia say is nonsense.
- People with schizophrenia cannot reliably report the effects of treatment or other things that happen to them.
- People with schizophrenia are completely unable to make rational decisions about their own lives (e.g. where to live).
- People with schizophrenia are unpredictable.
- People with schizophrenia cannot work.
- People with schizophrenia get progressively sicker all their lives.
- Schizophrenia is the parents' fault.

The stigma that attaches to schizophrenia extends beyond the individual with the illness to encompass everything and everyone associated with him or her. This includes the medications and other treatments that maybe used to control symptoms, family members (who are often wrongly considered to have caused the illness), other caregivers, health professionals who care for those with schizophrenia, and even the hospitals and other institutions in which those with schizophrenia are treated.

Extent of the stigma

It is clear that people with mental illness are highly stigmatized in the West. Branded as 'psychos' in popular parlance, they encounter discrimination in housing and employment (Miller and Dawson, 1965) and generate fear that they are dangerous. Citizens fight to exclude treatment facilities and living quarters for the mentally ill from residential neighbourhoods. According to a 1990 survey of the American public, the 'not in my backyard' phenomenon is a widespread obstacle to the community integration of people with mental illness (Robert Wood Johnson Foundation, 1990). The status afforded the mentally ill is the very lowest – lower than that of ex-convicts or the developmentally disabled (Tringo, 1970). According to one US survey, even after 5 years of normal living and hard work, an ex-mental patient is rated as less acceptable than an ex-convict (Lamy, 1966).

The agencies serving the mentally ill are tainted by association and mental health professionals themselves sometimes hold attitudes towards mental patients that are similar to those of the general public; they may even be more rejecting. In one study, mental hospital staff were considerably less likely than members of the public to take the trouble to mail a sealed, addressed letter which they believed to have been accidentally lost by a mental hospital patient (Page, 1980).

Tragically, people with mental illness themselves accept the stereotype of their own condition. Young patients in rural Ireland viewed 'spending time in the "madhouse" … as a permanent "fall from grace" similar to a loss of virginity' (Scheper-Hughes, 1979; p. 89). A number of studies have shown that mental patients are as negative in their opinions of mental illness as the general public (Giovannoni and Ullman, 1963; Manis *et al.*, 1963; Crumpton *et al.*, 1967). Some reports, indeed, indicate that mental patients are more rejecting of the mentally ill than are family members or hospital staff (Bentinck, 1967; Swanson and Spitzer, 1970).

In a comparison of attitudes towards the mentally ill at sites in four European countries: (people in Athens) Greece and (Naples) Italy, were more rejecting than those in Britain and Sweden. Most of the respondents in Greece and Italy felt that 'lack of will power' was a primary cause of mental illness and believed that the mentally ill were 'far more dangerous than most suppose' (Hall *et al.*, 1991).

Some individual factors are known to moderate stigma and improve public tolerance of the mentally ill. Younger and better educated people are usually more tolerant (Rabkin, 1980; Brockington *et al.*, 1993; Wolff, 1997). Prior contact with someone who suffers from mental illness decreases stigma and fear of dangerousness, as does knowledge of the person's living situation (Penn *et al.*, 1994). Those who do not perceive the mentally ill as violent are relatively tolerant (Link *et al.*, 1987; Penn *et al.*, 1994). Residential facilities for the mentally ill are better accepted in downtown, transient districts with low social cohesion, while they are less well accepted in single-family neighbourhoods (Trute and Segal, 1976).

A survey in England, Scotland and Wales (MORI, 1997) seemed to indicate an improvement in public attitudes towards schizophrenia, at least with regard to treatment possibilities and integration into the community. In this study, 59% of those surveyed felt that schizophrenia can be treated effectively while only 10% disagreed; only 18% said that they would not be willing to work alongside someone with schizophrenia while 54% disagreed; 12% felt that people with schizophrenia should live in institutions for the mentally ill, not in neighbourhood areas, while 64% disagreed; and, finally, 72% felt that, with careful support and appropriate treatment with modern medicines, people with schizophrenia can live successfully in the community. However, when questions about more personal issues were posed, the public's tolerance appears to change to a more neutral or negative feeling, with only 13% saying they would be happy if their son or daughter was going out with someone with schizophrenia, while 47% disagreed.

People with schizophrenia are often viewed differently in developing countries

A number of factors in developing countries result in greater tolerance, and continued family and community support for those with serious mental illness. In developing countries, persons with mental illness and schizophrenia have traditionally lived in the community and with their own families. In addition, large-scale institutionalization has not been a part of the mental health care system in these countries. Other factors contributing to greater tolerance and support are:

- the rural agrarian nature of the society;
- strong family system with filial affiliation;
- models for explaining the cause of the illness that are external (e.g. spirits) and are shared by community members;
- reversibility of behaviour including symptoms.

However, this situation could change with increasing urbanization, the influence of mass media, and the breakdown of family structure.

A number of studies in the 1970s and earlier found that a lower level of stigma was attached to mental disorder in developing countries and that those with mental illness were often better tolerated by families and were the object of less criticism and hostility. Among the Formosan tribes-men studied by Rin and Lin (1962), mental illness was free of stigma. Sinhalese families freely refer to their psychotic family members as pissu (crazy) and show no shame about it; tuberculosis in Sri Lanka was more stigmatizing than mental illness (Waxler, 1977).

The lower level of stigma in parts of the developing world may be a result of different folk-diagnostic practices. Throughout the non-industrial world, the features of psychosis are likely to be given a supernatural explanation (e.g. people with these symptoms may be considered the victims of witchcraft, shamans or spiritualists (Warner, 1974)). When urban and rural Yoruba with no formal education from Abeokuta in Nigeria were asked their opinions about profiles of mentally ill people, only 40% of those questioned thought the person described with symptoms of paranoid schizophrenia was mentally ill (Erinosho and Ayonrinde 1981), whereas nearly all Americans labelled the subject of this vignette as mentally ill (D'Arcy and Brockman, 1976). Only a fifth of uneducated Yorubans considered the person described with symptoms of simple schizophrenia to be mentally ill, versus three-quarters of American respondents (D'Arcy and Brockman, 1976). A third of the uneducated Yoruba would have been willing to marry the person with paranoid schizophrenia and more than half would have married the person with simple schizophrenia. However, when skilled workers from the area of Benin in mid-western Nigeria were asked their opinions about someone specifically labelled a 'nervous or mad person,' 16% thought that all such people should be shot and 31% believed that they should be expelled from the country. These educated Nigerians conceived of mad people as 'senseless, unkempt, aggressive and irresponsible' (Binitie, 1970).

The World Health Organization (WHO) multicentre study in four developing countries studied community attitudes using seven case vignettes in Columbia, India, Philippines and Sudan. This study found that the community differentiated the different disorders in terms of severity, treatability, marriagiability and desirability as neighbours (Wig *et al.*, 1980). The respondents placed greater emphasis on external behaviour rather than internal symptoms experienced by the individual.

Indian mental health professionals have conducted many studies on the attitude of the general public towards mental illness. Again, earlier studies found higher levels of tolerance than in developed countries. A survey of Indian professionals (Sathyavathi *et al.*, 1971) found that they were willing to interact with the mentally ill in various aspects of life and would not feel the need to conceal the illness of someone in their own family. Similarly, most adults in Vellore, India, when interviewed, were sympathetic towards mental patients and accepted modern treatment methods available in hospital (Verghese and Beig, 1974). The respondents expressed optimism about the outcome of treatment, especially if provided dearly in the course of the illness. However, nearly two-thirds of the respondents felt that the cure could be only partial and also opposed marital alliances with families in which there is a history of mental illness.

The authors of a WHO follow-up study of schizophrenia suggest that one of the factors contributing to the good outcome from schizophrenia in Cali, Colombia, is the 'high level of tolerance of relatives and friends for symptoms of mental disorder,' a factor that can help the 'readjustment to family life and work after discharge' (WHO, 1979). In an Indian 5-year follow-up study of persons with schizophrenia, 80% of families preferred that the person continue to stay with the family (ICMR, 1988). Another study found home care treatment for persons with schizophrenia was more accepted and less disruptive for families than hospital care (Pai and Kapur, 1983).

More recent findings, however, have shown that with increasing urbanization and the breakdown of traditional values and social structures, there has been a decline in tolerance for the mentally ill in industrializing parts of the developing world. In a review of public attitudes towards mental illness in New Delhi, India, Prabhu *et al.* (1984) concluded that 'the lay public, including the educated urban groups, are largely uninformed about the various aspects of mental health. The mentally ill are perceived as aggressive, violent and dangerous. There is a lack of awareness about the available facilities to treat the mentally ill and a pervasive defeatism exists about the possible outcome after therapy. There is a tendency to maintain social distance from the mentally ill and to reject them'.

It is clear that attitudes to the mentally ill vary from culture to culture and are influenced by the label that is applied to the person with psychosis.

REFERENCES – APPENDIX II

Bentinck, C. (1967). Opinions about mental illness held by patients and relatives. *Family Process*, **6**, 193–207.

Binitie, A.O. (1970). Attitude of educated Nigerians to psychiatric illness. *Acta Psychiatrica Scandinavica*, **46**, 391–398.

Brockington, I.F., Hall, P., Levings, J., *et al.* (1993). The community's tolerance of the mentally ill. *British Journal of Psychiatry*, **162**, 93–99.

D'Arcy, C. and Brockman, J. (1976). Changing public recognition of psychiatric symptoms? Blackfoot revisited. *Journal of Health Social Behaviour*, **17**, 302–310.

Crumpton, E., Weinstein, A.D., Acker, C.W., *et al.* (1967). How patients and normals see the mental patient. *Journal of Clinical Psychology*, **23**, 46–49.

Erinosho, O.A. and Ayonrinde, A. (1981). Educational background and attitude to mental illness among the Yoruba in Nigeria. *Human Relations*, **34**, 1–12.

Giovannoni, J.M. and Ullman, L.P. (1963). Conceptions of mental health held by psychiatric patients. *Journal of Clinical Psychology*, **19**, 398–400.

Hall, P., Brockington, I., Eisemann, C., Madianos, M., Maj, M. (1991). "Difficult to place" psychiatric patients. *British Journal of Psychiatry*, **302**, 1150.

Indian Council of Medical Research (ICMR). (1988). Multicentred collaborative study of factors associated with the cause and outcome of schizophrenia. New Delhi, India: ICMR.

Lamy, R.E. (1966). Social consequences of mental illness. *Journal Consulting Psychology*, **30**, 450–455.

Link, B.G., Cullen, F.T., Frank, J., *et al.* (1987). The social rejection of former mental patients: Understanding why labels matter. *American Journal of Sociology*, **92**, 1461–1500.

Manis, M., Houts, P.S. and Blake, J.B. (1963). Beliefs about mental illness as a function of psychiatric status and psychiatric hospitalization. *Journal of Abnormal and Social Psychology*, **67**, 226–233.

Miller, D. and Dawson, W.H. (1965). Effects of stigma on re-employment of ex-mental patients. *Mental Hygiene*, **49**, 281–287.

MORI. (1997). *Attitudes Toward Schizophrenia: A survey of public opinions*. Research study conducted by Fleishman Hillard Eli Lilly, September.

Page, S. (1980). Social responsiveness toward mental patients: the general public and others. *Canadian Journal of Psychiatry*, **25**, 242–246.

Pai, S. and Kapur, R.L. (1983). Evaluation of home care treatment for schizophrenic patients. *Acta Psychiatrica Scandinavica*, **67**, 80–88.

Penn, D.L., Guynan, K., Daily, T., *et al.* (1994). Dispelling the stigma of schizophrenia: what sort of information is best? *Schizophrenia Bulletin*, **20**, 567–578.

Prabhu, G.C., Raghuram, A., Verma, N., *et al.* (1984). Public attitudes toward mental illness: a review. *NIMHANS Journal*, **2**, 1–14.

Rabkin, J.G. (1980). Determinants of public attitudes about mental illness: summary of the research literature, presented at the *National Institute of Mental Health Conference on Stigma Toward the Mentally Ill*, Rockville, Maryland, January 24–25.

Rin, H. and Lin, T. (1962). Mental illness among Formosan aborigines as compared with the Chinese in Taiwan. *Journal of Mental Science*, **108**, 134–146.

Robert Wood Johnson Foundation. (1990). *Public Attitudes Toward People with Chronic Mental Illness*. New Jersey, The Robert Wood Johnson Foundation Program on Chronic Mental Illness, April.

Sathyavathi, K., Dwarki, B.R. and Murthy, H.N. (1971). Conceptions of mental health. *Transactions of All India Institute of Mental Health*, **11**, 37–49.

Scheper-Hughes, N. (1979). *Saints, Scholars and Schizophrenics: Mental Illness in Rural Ireland*. Berkeley, University of California Press, 89.

Swanson, R.M. and Spitzer, S.P. (1970). Stigma and the psychiatric patient career. *Journal of Health Social Behaviour*, **11**, 44–51.

Tringo, J.L. (1970). The hierarchy of preference towards disability groups. *Journal of Special Education*, **4**, 295–306.

Trute, B. and Segal, S.P. (1976). Census tract predictors and the social integration of sheltered care residents. *Social Psychiatry*, **11**, 153–161.

Verghese, A. and Beig, A. (1974). Public attitude towards mental illness: the Vellore study. *Indian Journal of Psychiatry*, **16**, 8–18.

Warner, R. (1974). *Recovery from Schizophrenia: Psychiatry and Political Economy*, 2nd edn. London, Routledge.

Waxler, N.E. (1977). Is mental illness cured in traditional societies? A theoretical analysis. *Culture Medicine and Psychiatry*, **1**, 233–253.

Wig, N.N., Suleiman, M.A., Routledge, R., *et al.* (1980). Community reactions to mental disorders: a key informant study in three developing countries. *Acta Psychiatrica Scandinavica*, **61**, 111–126.

Wolff, G. (1997). Attitudes of the media and the public. In Leff, J., ed. *Care in the Community: Illusion or Reality?* New York, Wiley.

World Health Organization. (1979). *Schizophrenia: An International Follow-up Study.* Chichester, England, Wiley.

Appendix III
Presentation evaluation

(Used in Calgary, Canada to assess presentations of the Partnership Programme)

We would appreciate your time in answering the following few questions about the presentation. Your responses will help us evaluate whether we are meeting our goals and will help us to improve our performance.

1 Has your knowledge about schizophrenia improved as a result of this presentation?
   ❑ Not at all   ❑ Somewhat   ❑ Considerably

2 Has this presentation changed your attitude towards people with schizophrenia?
   ❑ My attitude has become more positive
   ❑ My attitude has not changed
   ❑ My attitude has become more negative

3 Has your knowledge about other mental illnesses improved as a result of this presentation?
   ❑ Not at all   ❑ Somewhat   ❑ Considerably

4 Has this presentation changed your attitude towards people with a mental illness?
   ❑ My attitude has become more positive
   ❑ My attitude has not changed
   ❑ My attitude has become more negative

5 What part of this presentation had the most benefit for you?
   _____
   _____
   _____

6 What part of this presentation would you improve?
   _____
   _____
   _____

7 Do you think that you will now act differently towards people with a mental illness as a result of this presentation? Please explain.

_____

_____

_____

8 To further help us with our analysis, will you tell us how old you are?
 _____ years

9 Are you?
 ❏ Male   ❏ Female

10 What are the first three digits of your postal code? ____ ____ ____

Community pre/post-survey

Hello, this is (name) calling for the Calgary Regional Health Authority. We are doing a short 10 min survey about mental health. Could I speak to someone in the household 15 years of age or older?

In which of the following categories does your age fall? Read list

Age:
❏ 15–29 years old
❏ 30–59 years old
❏ 60 years of age or older

Gender:
❏ Male   ❏ Female

Region:
❏ Calgary area
❏ Drumheller area

1 In the past 6 months, have you seen, read or heard any advertising or promotions about schizophrenia?
 ❏ Yes   ❏ No

(1a) If yes, where did you see, read or heard the advertisement or promotions?

_____

_____

Do not read. Record all responses. Probe with anywhere else? (List up to three responses)
❏ Television
❏ Radio

❑ *Calgary Herald* (newspaper)
❑ *Calgary Sun* (newspaper)
❑ *Calgary Mirror* (newspaper)
❑ *Calgary Rural Times* (newspaper)
❑ *Drumheller Mail* (newspaper)
❑ Other newspaper
❑ Newsletters from community leagues, non-profit organizations, etc.
❑ Magazine
❑ Brochure/pamphlet
❑ Poster
❑ Outdoor billboards
❑ Busboard/advertising on the bus
❑ Other media
❑ Don't remember/don't know

2 In the past 6 months, have you seen, read or heard anything in the news about people with schizophrenia?
❑ Yes   ❑ No

(2a) If yes, could you tell me how the person with schizophrenia was described?

_____

_____

Do not read. Probe with anything else? (List up to three responses)
❑ Violent or dangerous to others
❑ Committing a crime
❑ Homeless
❑ A public nuisance
❑ Dishevelled in appearance or dirty
❑ Suffering from symptoms, such as hearing voices or speaking to self
❑ Suicidal or depressed
❑ A victim of crime
❑ The victim of serious illness (e.g. requiring medical treatment)
❑ In need of better treatment or support systems
❑ Involved in research
❑ Other positive description
❑ Other negative description
❑ Don't remember/don't know

3 Do you or have you ever worked as an employee in an agency that provides services to people with emotional problems or mental illnesses?
❑ Yes   ❑ No

4   Have you or someone you know ever been treated for an emotional problem or a mental illness?
    ❏ Yes   ❏ No   ❏ Not sure

    (4a) If yes, was that … Read list
    ❏ Yourself
    ❏ Spouse/child
    ❏ Other relation
    ❏ Friend
    ❏ Acquaintance
    ❏ Co-worker

5   Have you or someone you know ever been treated for schizophrenia?
    ❏ Yes   ❏ No   ❏ Not sure

    (5a) If yes, was that … *Read list*
    ❏ Yourself
    ❏ Spouse/child
    ❏ Other relation
    ❏ Friend
    ❏ Acquaintance
    ❏ Co-worker

6   Schizophrenia can touch the lives of many people, often through close friends or relatives, but also through work, volunteerism or life in general. To what extent does schizophrenia affect your life? *Read list*
    ❏ Not at all
    ❏ Somewhat
    ❏ Quite a bit
    ❏ All the time, that is, you deal with it almost daily

7   To the best of your knowledge, what causes schizophrenia? *Do not read. Probe with anything else? Record all responses* (List up to three responses)
    ❏ Physical abnormalities in the brain
    ❏ Chemical imbalance in the brain
    ❏ Brain disease
    ❏ Virus during pregnancy
    ❏ Genetical inheritance
    ❏ Other biological factor
    ❏ Poor upbringing by parents
    ❏ Physical abuse
    ❏ Drug or alcohol abuse

❑ Stress (such as losing a job, social stress)
❑ Traumatic event or shock (e.g. assault, death, and accident)
❑ Poverty
❑ General breakdown in social values
❑ Possession by evil spirits. God's punishment
❑ Other factors
❑ The exact causes are unknown
❑ Don't know

8 All things considered, do you believe people with schizophrenia … *Read statement …*
(1) Frequently (2) Often (3) Rarely or (4) Never
❑ Can be successfully treated outside of the hospital in the community
❑ Tend to be mentally retarded or of lower intelligence
❑ Hear voices telling them what to do
❑ Need prescription drugs to control their symptoms
❑ Can be successfully treated without drugs using psychotherapy or social interventions
❑ Are a public nuisance due to panhandling, poor hygiene or odd behaviour
❑ Suffer from split or multiple personalities
❑ Can be seen talking to themselves or shouting in city streets
❑ Can work in regular jobs
❑ Are dangerous to the public because of violent behaviour

9 To the best of your knowledge, what per cent of the population suffers from schizophrenia? *Round off percentage*
❑ _____ per cent
❑ Don't know

10 Please tell me how you would feel in each of the following situations using the scale …
(1) Definitely (2) Probably (3) Probably not (4) Definitely not
Read each statement. Record one answer per statement.
❑ Would you feel afraid to have a conversation with someone who has schizophrenia?
❑ Would you be upset or disturbed about working on the same job with someone who has schizophrenia?
❑ Would you be able to maintain a friendship with someone who has schizophrenia?

❑ Would you feel upset or disturbed about rooming with someone who has schizophrenia?

❑ Would you feel ashamed if people knew someone in your family has been diagnosed with schizophrenia?

❑ Would you marry someone with schizophrenia?

11 How would you feel about having a group home for six to eight people with schizophrenia in your neighbourhood? Would you be … *Read list*

❑ In favour

❑ Opposed

❑ In different, that is, it doesn't matter

Finally just a few questions to help us classify and better understand all of the survey results.

_____

_____

12 On average, how many hours of television a week do you watch?

_____ ## Hours watched

13 And what age did you turn on your last birthday?

_____ ##

14 What is the highest level of education you have completed? Would it be … *Read list*

❑ Elementary or up to and including Grade 6

❑ Junior high or Grades 7–9

❑ High school or Grades 10–13

❑ College or technical school

❑ University

15 In which country were you born?

_____

What is your postal code? ____ ____ ____ ____ ____ ____

Well, that's the last of my questions. Thanks so much for answering this survey. We really appreciate the time you took.

Appendix IV
ER recommendations and survey

(Includes surveys done with Alberta, Canada hospitals to evaluate emergency room (ER) treatment on those with schizophrenia, and recommendations submitted)

ER policies and procedures affecting those with schizophrenia

For the Local Advisory Committee of the World Psychiatric Association (WPA) Global Project on Stigma and Schizophrenia
23 November, 1998

Sub-Committee on health care professionals target group

Gus Thompson, PhD	University of Alberta and Calgary, Chair
Roger Bland, MB	University of Alberta
Marian Ewing, RPN	Health Authority #5
Michelle Misurelli	Schizophrenia Society of Alberta
Beth Evans, BA	Provincial Mental Health Advisory Board
Julio Arboleda Flórez, MD, PhD	Queen's University
Laurie Beverly, MN	Calgary Regional Health Authority
Ruth Dickson, MD	Peter Lougheed Centre

Prepared by:
Gus Thompson
Roger Bland
Marian Ewing

Comments on this discussion paper can be directed to:
Dr Gus Thompson, Department of Psychiatry, University of Alberta, Edmonton, Alberta T6G 2G3.
Phone (403) 492-8753. E-mail to: Gus.Thompson@ualberta.ca

The questionnaire

The questionnaire was designed to elicit information on matters thought by the Sub-Committee to be highly relevant to the treatment of people with schizophrenia. These included privacy, security (for patients and staff), policies on patient rights

and the use of restraints, staff training in mental health and crisis management, waiting times and patient/family satisfaction with services. Questionnaires
were completed by the respondents at their leisure and mailed or faxed to the
research team.

Privacy/security

The responses suggest that the ERs at the Peter Lougheed Centre and the Rocky
View General Hospital have adequate rooms for the provision of secure and private
services for the mentally ill patients but the Drumheller General Hospital and the
Foothills Medical Centre do not. Upcoming planning and development activities
may improve the situation at the Foothills Medical Centre.

All the Calgary hospitals report having good access to security staff but the
Drumheller General Hospital appears to have such staff only available during
restricted hours and without ready access in any case.

Patient rights

Policies governing patient rights are formalized for all the Calgary hospitals, but
apparently not at the Drumheller General Hospital. In no case is a statement of
rights presented to patients with schizophrenia (or their families) as a matter of
course. The Peter Lougheed Centre will provide this upon patient request.

The Calgary hospitals have a policy on the use of restraints, but the opinion is
mixed among the respondents for the Drumheller General Hospital.

Training

All the ERs in the Calgary hospitals reportedly provide onsite psychiatric staff
who had received specific training in the handling of mental health emergencies.
However, these individuals are not available at all times. For the Peter Lougheed
Centre, such staff are onsite for 60 h/week (1 week + 168 h). The figure is 112 h for
both the Rocky View General Hospital and the Foothills Medical Centre. In all
cases, specialists are on call at all times. Continuing Medical Education (CME) in
this topic area is not required, although some is offered in Calgary.

ER staff, although not always formally trained in psychiatry/mental health will
have received some expertise in the handling of mental health crises as part of
their formal education. They may be selected for this attribute by the Calgary
hospitals who also require in service in this area. However, the respondents for
the Drumheller General Hospital provided the opinion that their staff are not well
prepared. Notably, in service is not required at the Drumheller General Hospital.

Satisfaction

According to the respondents, none of the hospitals have data that would deal with the question of whether psychiatric patients have to wait longer for services than others, although a study is about to be conducted in Calgary. Several respondents noted that all patients are treated equally, and there should thus be no differences.

Similarly, no data were presented that reflected client satisfaction with services. The consensus appeared to be that no such data exists, although one respondent noted that a number of 'local' studies might have been conducted in the past.

Planned improvements

The aforementioned Foothills Medical Centre planning review notwithstanding, none of the respondents noted the existence of any firm plans to address any of the ER issues noted above.

Additional respondent comments

Among the Calgary respondents, there was a stated belief that ER psychiatry is neglected to some degree by 'mainstream' psychiatry/mental health and marginalized by the ER departments. The resource issue that was identified pertained to 'backing up' in ERs due to non-ER beds being full. One respondent pointed out that members of her psychiatric ER team are 'excellent'. The Drumheller General Hospital respondents almost unanimously identified a need for more staff and more training.

Discussion and recommendations

While the differences across the hospitals are important and interesting, in many aspects, they are not the most important issue in the long run. Rather, what is important is whether or not psychiatric patients in emergency departments are treated appropriately. A key to this is the adoption of acceptable standards and practices by each hospital with an ER. Perhaps the best way to achieve this is to have suitable questions added to the accreditation process that each hospital in Alberta is engaged in on a regular basis. To this end, preliminary discussions have been held with the Canadian Council on Health Services Accreditation (CCHSA), which is the accrediting body that surveys all Canadian hospitals. Furthermore, appropriate staff from both the Drumheller and Calgary Regional Health Authorities have requested copies of this report as an aid to their approach to future accreditation reviews. In support of this, the items from our ER survey have been recast in the CCHSA questionnaire format in order to facilitate this kind of use.

It should be noted that we received very good support and cooperation from the ER staff at all the hospitals that we approached. They would be very interested in feedback from us on this activity.

Thus, our recommendations are:

1 That the ER guidelines as formulated in be sent to the CCHSA for consideration for adoption by that body and for inclusion in their survey instrument.
2 That we provide copies of our findings and recommendation to the participating ER Directors in Drumheller and Calgary, the Managers of Patient Care for the Calgary Regional Health Authority and Health Authority #5, and the Provincial Mental Health Advisory Board.

Questionnaire

Are your ER medical staff trained in managing mental health crises?

- Are they required to participate in CME in this area?
- How does this compare with requirements, training and qualification in other areas of medicine?

Are your other staff (e.g. nurses) trained in managing mental health emergencies?

- If trained, how did they receive the training?
- Is there any in-service requirement in this field?

If you have data on whether wait times differ in any way from those with other illnesses or conditions, please provide the most recent results.

If you have data on patient (mental health) and family satisfaction with your ER services, please provide a copy of the most recent results. Please include data, if possible, drawn from patients with other illnesses. Is such data collected on a regular basis

Do you have plans for any changes in the above areas?

Do you have any comments pertaining to the care of the mentally ill in emergency departments?

Proposed summary accreditation guidelines

Prepared by

The Sub-Committee on Health Care Professionals Target Group for the Local Advisory Committee of the WPA Global Project on Stigma and Schizophrenia

Gus Thompson, Chair

Roger Bland

Michelle Misurelli

Marian Ewing
Beth Evans
Julio Arboleda-Flórez
Laurie Beverly
Ruth Dickson

Special guidelines for patients with a mental illness

		Organization's rating				Surveyor's rating			
		N	M	P	S	N	M	P	S
P1.0	The examination and interview process and space are adequate for the safety, security and privacy of patients and staff								
P1.1	There are enough private interview rooms available to ensure privacy during interviews in most situations								
P1.2	Interview rooms are secure								
P1.3	Security staff are available on a timely, as needed, basis								
P1.4	There is a policy in place governing the use of restraints								

Index